Holding On to Home

The Johns Hopkins Series in Contemporary Medicine and Public Health

Also of Interest in This Series:

William Halsey Barker, M.D., *Adding Life to Years: Organized Geriatrics Services in Great Britain and Implications for the United States*

Dorothy H. Coons, ed., *Specialized Dementia Care Units*

Carl Eisdorfer, Ph.D., M.D., David A. Kessler, M.D., J.D., and Abby N. Spector, M.M.H.S., eds., *Caring for the Elderly: Reshaping Health Policy*

Nancy L. Mace, ed., *Dementia Care: Patient, Family, and Community*

Vincent Mor, Ph.D., David S. Greer, M.D., and Robert Kastenbaum, Ph.D., eds., *The Hospice Experiment*

William G. Weissert, Jennifer M. Elston, Elise J. Bolda, William N. Zelman, Elizabeth Mutran, and Anne B. Mangum, *Adult Day Care: Findings from a National Survey*

Holding On to Home

**Designing Environments
for People with Dementia**

Uriel Cohen

Gerald D. Weisman

School of Architecture and Urban Planning

University of Wisconsin–Milwaukee

The Johns Hopkins University Press
Baltimore & London

This book was sponsored by the Retirement Research Foundation, with additional support from the Health Facilities Research Program of the American Institute of Architects/ Association of Collegiate Schools of Architecture, and the Design Arts Program of the National Endowment for the Arts.

Principal Research and Design Assistants: Kristen Day, Keya Ray, and William Robison

The Johns Hopkins University Press
701 West 40th Street
Baltimore, Maryland 21211
The Johns Hopkins Press Ltd., London

The paper used in this book meets the minimum requirements of American National Standard for Information Sciences—Permanence of Paper for Printed Library Materials, ANSI Z39.48-1984.

Library of Congress Cataloging-in-Publication Data

Cohen, Uriel.
    Holding on to home: designing environments for people with dementia / Uriel Cohen and Gerald D. Weisman.
        p.   cm. — (The Johns Hopkins series in contemporary medicine and public health)
    Includes bibliographical references.
    Includes index.
    ISBN 0-8018-4069-4 (alk. paper)
    1. Alzheimer's disease—Patients—Dwellings. 2. Senile dementia—Patients—Dwellings. 3. Long-term care facilities—Design and construction.   I. Weisman, Gerald D.   II. Title.   III. Series.
    [DNLM: 1. Alzheimer's Disease. 2. Environment Design. 3. Facility Design and Construction.   WM 27.1 C678h]
RC523.C653   1991
362.1'96831—dc20
DNLM/DLC   90-4785

Contents

Contents

Preface

Holding On to Home is about people with dementia and the environments in which they live. It seeks to expand our appreciation and understanding of the potential influence of architectural settings on the behavior and quality of life of people with dementia and of those who care for them. *Holding On to Home* explores relationships between architecture and behavior in terms of both theory and application, linking conceptual issues surrounding the care of people with dementia with innovative and practical approaches to the use of the physical environment as a therapeutic tool. While the progression of Alzheimer's disease and related dementias is inexorable, environmental interventions can be utilized to mediate some of the negative consequences. *Holding On to Home* also endeavors to expand our conceptualization of facilities for people with dementia, viewing them as points along a continuum, from residence in the community to specialized units within settings for long-term care; emphasis is placed upon the creation of new facility types at selected points along this continuum. While people with dementia and their environmental needs are the point of departure and primary focus of *Holding On to Home*, attention is also directed to the problems and needs of family caregivers, health and social service professionals, and facility administrators, as well as the concerns of architects, designers, and planners of environments for this population. To accomplish these multiple goals, *Holding On to Home* does not prescribe specific solutions. Rather, our intentions are to generate and present a clear formulation of the problem and to serve as a source of flexible ideas and generalizable directions for decision making.

It must be recognized from the outset that very little of the research into Alzheimer's disease explores linkages to the physical environment. Most research activities are directed toward either medical and biological issues, such as possible causes of the disease, or social/organizational concerns, such as caregiver burden. Of the limited research that directly explores the role of the environment as a therapeutic tool, much is experiential or anecdotal. Therefore, most of the recommendations advanced in *Holding On to Home* are, of necessity, extrapolations from existing research and experience. In the strong tradition of action research, they are presented as hypotheses deserving and indeed requiring further investigation.

Holding On to Home creates linkages between the problems of people with dementia and unique and sensitive solutions, emphasizing the environmental components of each. The organization of the book therefore parallels the facility delivery process—the typical sequence of activities required in the planning and creation of any environment for people with dementia. *Holding On to Home* begins with an introductory section that reviews the basic assumptions and values that underlie the entire book. Chapter 1 places basic problems of people with dementia and their caregivers into an environmental context and presents a set of therapeutic goals to guide subsequent planning, programming, and design decisions. Chapters 2 to 5 introduce a series of principles for the planning and design of facilities for people with dementia. Each of these principles comprises a synopsis of the needs to be met, the goals that must be realized, and a set of design and planning concepts, with examples that illustrate characteristics of appropriate solutions to the problems. These principles are integrated and illustrated through the design of five prototypical facilities presented in chapter 6. Finally, in chapter 7, the book concludes with a set of questions for the evaluation of environments for people with dementia.

It is our hope that *Holding On to Home* will contribute to a better understanding of the therapeutic potential of the physical environment and a more informed process of planning and design. A larger goal, which we share with all of those individuals upon whose work this book builds, is the creation of more supportive environments and an enhanced quality of life for people with dementia and their caregivers.

Acknowledgments

The preparation and production of *Holding On to Home* has been a complex effort involving many people, all of whom have contributed in important ways. An initial grant from the Health Facilities Research Program (HFRP) of the American Institute of Architects (AIA)/Association of Collegiate Schools of Architecture (ACSA) started us on the path that led to *Holding On to Home*; Richard McCommons of ACSA, Earle Kennett, Director of the HFRP, and Tib Tusler and Howard Juster of the AIA Committee on Architecture for Health were all central in launching this effort.

A grant from the Design Arts Program of the National Endowment for the Arts (NEA) made possible the translation of principles for planning and design into the prototypical designs presented in chapter 6. This NEA support has extended the scope of *Holding On to Home* and opened up new directions for design guidance.

Primary support for the development of *Holding On to Home* has come from the Retirement Research Foundation of Park Ridge, Illinois. Brian Hofland, Vice President of the foundation, provided valuable suggestions during the shaping of our project and introduced us to the highly relevant contributions of a number of researchers in gerontology.

Over the past two years, staff members hosted our visits at more than twenty sites, responded to our lengthy interviews, and provided valuable observations and suggestions; we express our gratitude to all of them. M. Powell Lawton provided both access to the Philadelphia Geriatric Center (PGC) and important insights regarding aging and environment research based upon two decades of pioneering research at PGC. Dorothy Coons, Maggie Calkins, and Paul Windley were generous with their time and observations. Barbara Keyes, Carol Goodman, and Susan Berry of the Wisconsin Alzheimer's Association provided invaluable help and information throughout the project. Thanks also go to the many architects, administrators, and Alzheimer's caregivers who reviewed an early draft of the design guidelines and particularly to the participants in our intensive three-day workshop for their critical and insightful review comments and ideas.

David Hoglund of Perkins, Geddis & Eastman Architects provided handsome illustrations and helpful suggestions. Ken Hanson and the staff of Hanson Graphic contributed to the visual quality of *Holding On to Home*. Krista Elich, Suzanne Larson, and Carolyn Lookabill were instrumental in arranging for many of the photographs. Our heartfelt thanks go to Pat and Jerry Schmidt and to Frances, Anna, and Louisa at Marina View Manor and to their families for sharing their lives with us and for the compelling photos that resulted. Thanks also go to Tom Bamberger, Robert Glick, Susie Post, and David Denemark, the photographers responsible for these images.

More than a dozen individuals have contributed their time and efforts as members of our project staff over the past two years. Victoria Steiner, Joseph Rand, and Richard Toyne made important contributions in the launching of our original AIA/ACSA project. James Dicker, AIA, and George Meyer, AIA, took the lead in developing prototypical designs. Kate Reed was an ever patient editor. Setsuko Sasaki, Somkeit C. Thumrong, Somkiat Khouvong, Sungkin Chiu, and Mary Gorman provided assistance with graphics and illustrations; Barbara Cooper provided much of the research and writing on the

Acknowledgements

nature of Alzheimer's disease. Kristen Day, Keya Ray, and William Robison have, for the past year, worked tirelessly as our colleagues, contributing insights, ideas, and enthusiasm. The Department of Architecture, the Center for Architectural and Urban Planning Research, and the Graduate School of the University of Wisconsin–Milwaukee all provided us with financial, logistical, and moral support. Finally, we would like to thank Wendy Harris, medical editor, Linda Forlifer, manuscript editor, and Kimberly Johnson, production editor, of the Johns Hopkins University Press, for taking us and this book through the production cycle and for superb editing.

Holding On To Home

Overleaf: Hanson Graphic; Ernest Gooding, photographed by Tom Bamberger

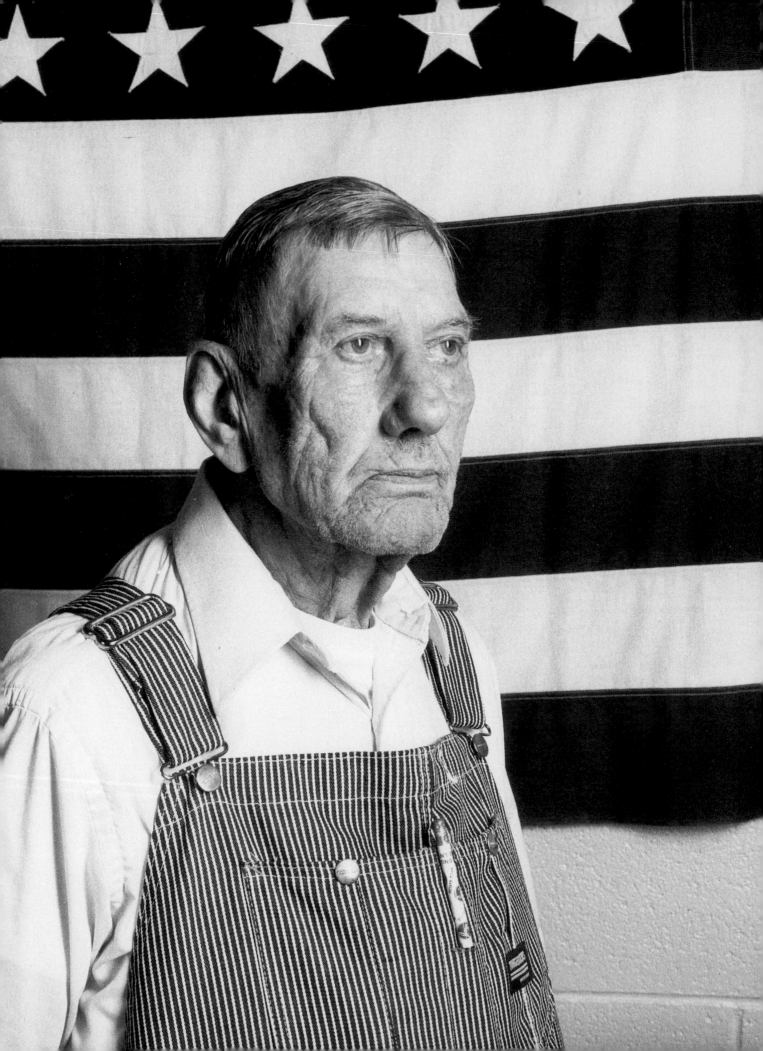

Introduction

Holding On to Home is about Alzheimer's disease and environmental design. These seem, at the outset, to be two disparate topics, and it might be asked what possible relationship they bear to each other. This introduction provides only a brief answer to this important question. In the following seven chapters linkages between Alzheimer's disease and environmental design are more fully developed and the potentially significant therapeutic role of the physical setting is clarified.

The goals and contents of *Holding On to Home* rest on four fundamental premises. First, the role of the architectural environment need not and should not be limited to the mere provision of physical shelter. Thoughtfully designed architectural environments represent potentially valuable, albeit typically underutilized, therapeutic resources in the care of people with dementia. Conversely, it has been argued (Coons 1985, 13) that many of the behaviors attributed to Alzheimer's disease are, in part, a consequence of countertherapeutic settings.

Second, the physical settings occupied by people with dementia do not exist in isolation; rather, they are integral parts of a larger, complex system and must operate in concert with the social and organizational dimensions of this larger system. Thus, *Holding On to Home* is organized around a *conceptual model* that reflects the interaction of architectural, social, behavioral, and organizational variables.

Third, *Holding On to Home* places great value in the *residential* qualities of environments for people with dementia. Many such facilities, while well intentioned, do not—as a consequence of their medical or institutional characteristics—serve the best interests of people with dementia. To the extent possible, all therapeutic settings should "hold on" to the attributes of home. The following section, "Linking Alzheimer's Disease and Environmental Design," reviews both theoretical and empirical support for the therapeutic potential of the physical setting, presents the conceptual model around which this book is structured, and further develops the concept of "residential" quality.

Finally, the development of facilities for people with dementia is never simple. If such facilities are to provide the kinds of therapeutic benefits alluded to above, there must be a thoughtfully considered and systematic planning process. For this reason, a model of the basic phases of the *facility delivery process* (including preparation, planning, programming, design, and evaluation) serves as the framework for chapters 1 to 7 of *Holding On to Home* and is presented in the section entitled "The Facility Development Process." This introduction concludes with a brief consideration of the costs of facility development and the construction process.

Linking Alzheimer's Disease and Environmental Design

The Therapeutic Potential of the Physical Environment

The architectural environment can have a significant influence on the quality of life of people with dementia and their caregivers.

Therapeutic environments can slow the decline expected over time in the functional abilities of people with dementia.

The role of the architectural environment in therapeutic interventions for people with dementia has traditionally been quite limited. Interventions are defined and implemented in social, medical, and organizational terms, with architectural/environmental factors limited to concerns of hygiene or esthetics. However, study of the reciprocal relationships between people and their total environment over the past several decades demonstrates that the architectural setting is more than a background variable and may exert significant influence on the behavior and quality of life of both individuals and groups.

The study of environment-behavior relationships has emerged as an important area of inquiry in both the planning and design professions (Lang 1987) and the behavioral sciences (Gifford 1987). Within gerontology, study of the relationships between the behavior of older people and the settings they occupy—characterized by Lawton as "the environmental psychology of later life" (1987, 340)—has flourished as an approach to theory development, empirical research, and application in areas such as housing. Lawton, who has played a central role in the evolution and maturation of this work, also cautions that, despite much enthusiasm and energy, the emergence of hard data that can guide planning and design decisions has been slow. This is certainly the case for that subset of research that deals with the planning and design of environments for people with dementia.

Nevertheless, there are strong empirical and theoretical justifications behind efforts to utilize the therapeutic potential of the physical setting in the provision of care for people with dementia. Several studies assessing the effects of changes in the physical setting on people with dementia carried out by Lawton and associates were reviewed by Lawton (1981). A small-scale remodeling effort undertaken in a long-term care facility resulted in the creation of six single bedrooms plus adjacent semipublic spaces. Residents both took advantage of this new-found opportunity for privacy and increased the number of occasions on which they were observed outside their bedrooms (Lawton, Liebowitz & Charon 1970). Two pilot studies examined the effect of environmental modifications on a psychiatric geriatric population (Fraser 1978, Stahler, Frazer & Rappaport 1984). Rearrangement of furnishings and introduction of materials for recreation and reading resulted in some social gains and a decrease in pathological behavior. In a pioneering demonstration and research project, Lawton, Fulcomer, and Kleban (1984) compared the behavior of severely impaired, elderly residents of a nursing home before and after transfer to the Weiss Institute, a new facility designed in response to their environmental needs (fig. I.1). Results indicate that, despite expected decline in mea-

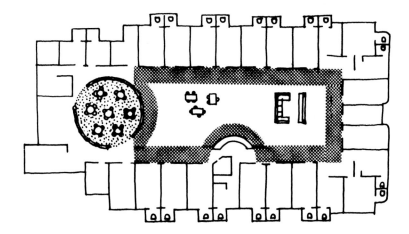

Figure I.1
A facility designed in response to the environmental needs of people with dementia. (The Weiss Institute, Philadelphia Geriatric Center.)

sures of basic competence, there was not a corresponding decline in more pliable behavioral variables. "Even more remarkably, in five instances improvement occurred, and in only one instance was there a significant decline. This pattern of findings . . . confirms the presence of a clear prosthetic effect, to the point where the direction of a decline was reversed in some instances to become improvement" (p. 751). More recently, a longitudinal study of a special care unit conducted by Benson et al. (1987) indicated improvements in mental and emotional status and in basic functions of daily living twelve months after admission to the unit.

A major research/demonstration project undertaken by the Institute of Gerontology at the University of Michigan created Wesley Hall, a special living unit for eleven people with severe memory loss (Coons 1985). Along with intensive training of staff, a number of modifications were made in the physical setting; these included the introduction of softer and more domestic finishes and lighting and the provision of private resident rooms and a den, living room, dining room, and kitchen as part of the Wesley Hall unit. Staff observations indicated positive resident response to therapeutic interventions designed to reduce problem behaviors such as night wandering, incontinence, and combativeness.

Theoretical support for the therapeutic role of the physical setting comes from several sources. Most prominent is the environmental docility hypothesis promulgated by Lawton and Nahemow (Lawton 1970, Lawton & Nahemow 1973), which posits that "limitations in health, cognitive skills, ego strength, status, social role performance, or degree of cultural evolution will tend to heighten the docility of the person in the face of environmental constraints and influences" (Lawton 1970, 40). Thus, people with dementia, who often experience impairments of the kinds described by Lawton, may be particularly vulnerable to environmental influences. Conversely, even modest modifications in the environment which serve to reduce what Lawton and Nahemow characterized as the "press" or demand characteristics of the environment may yield significant improvements in both adaptive behavior and affect. At least some clinically based dementia research (Hall & Buckwalter 1986) draws similar conclusions regarding the importance of conscious regulation of the

People with dementia may be especially responsive to even modest changes in their environment.

demand characteristics of the environment, particularly in terms of sensory and social stimulation.

In summary, there is both empirical and theoretical support for the positive role of the physical setting in the care of people with dementia. Data suggest that modification of traditional room and unit layouts, along with complementary modifications in the organizational environment, can slow or in some cases even reverse the decline over time expected in the behavior of people with dementia. Such findings seem to be consistent with Lawton's "environmental docility hypothesis," which suggests that even modest changes in the environments of people of reduced competence may have significant positive consequences.

The Environment as a Complex Setting

Any environment, as we experience it, reflects the interaction of architectural, organizational, and social factors.

The research reviewed above strongly suggests that the physical setting can indeed have a therapeutic role in the care of people with dementia. It demonstrates with equal clarity that the physical setting, by itself, rarely has a direct and deterministic effect upon patterns of human behavior (Ohta & Ohta, 1988). While the primary goal of *Holding On to Home* is to provide guidance for the planning and design of physical settings for people with dementia, architectural variables should not and cannot be considered in isolation. Whether a person with dementia will experience an environment as sufficiently private, comfortable, or stimulating is a consequence not only of building design but also of organizational policy and the behaviors and attitudes of others using the setting. Thus, the environment inhabited by people with dementia may usefully be viewed as a complex system comprising organizational, social, and physical components that interact in multiple ways (Moos & Lemke 1984). *Holding On to Home* conceptualizes this person-environment system in terms of a five-part framework (fig. I.2).

Figure I.2
A conceptual framework for the organization of the person-environment system.

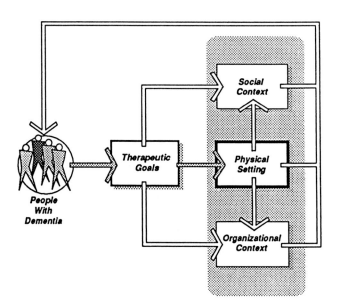

First and foremost are *people with dementia,* defined in terms of the physical, functional, and emotional capabilities and needs characteristic of their disease. As preparation, chapter 1 provides background material on dementia and profiles two people with Alzheimer's disease and their caregivers.

In response to the nature and needs of people with dementia, many authors formulate goals—such as "preservation of dignity or independence"—judged to be therapeutic. Such goals, although abstract in themselves, can provide decision makers with a general sense of guidance and direction for planning and design. A set of such *therapeutic goals,* presented in chapter 1, provides the foundation for the principles for planning and design in chapters 2 to 5.

The final three components of this conceptual model are the *organizational, social, and physical environments* within which people with dementia find themselves. The organizational component is conceptualized in terms of the policies and programs of long-term care facilities, group homes, or day care centers. The social component is represented by neighbors or fellow residents, as well as family and friends who serve critically important roles as caregivers. Finally, the architectural component is defined in terms of the experiential qualities or attributes of environments for people with dementia, the spatial organization of such environments, and the individual rooms and activity areas of which they are composed.

As represented in figure I.2, therapeutic goals—such as "the maintenance of ties to the healthy and familiar"—are shaped by the nature and needs of people with dementia. Such goals, in turn, help to define the organizational, social, and physical characteristics of the environment. A physical design response to the goal of maintaining ties to the healthy and familiar might include the use of residential furnishings, carpeting, and wallpaper in a group home for people with dementia to create positive associations with the family homes in which they previously lived. Such residential qualities may ease the transition to a new setting, contribute to residents' sense of comfort, and encourage visitation from family members. In this way, the physical setting, along with a carefully designed organizational environment, can contribute to the realization of desired therapeutic goals and have a positive effect on the lives of people with dementia.

The Concept of Home

Although there has been limited study of the psychosocial consequences of the environments in which people with dementia live (Lawton 1987), there is one theme that clearly permeates this literature and that provides both the title and the theme of *Holding On to Home.* This is the theme of "homelike," "domestic," or "noninstitutional" environments and the therapeutic importance of creating such settings for people with dementia.

The Wesley Hall research/demonstration project is probably the clearest reflection of this emphasis on the "homelike" qualities of settings for people with dementia (fig. I.3). Wesley Hall endeavored to erase those features of the physical and organizational environments that were viewed as "constant reminders of sickness and institutional living" (Coons 1987, 34). There was no intercom. Instead of a nursing station, staff kept records at a small table in the kitchen. Staff members wore regular clothes instead of uniforms. To the ex-

A true sense of home is created through opportunities to personalize one's environment and have some measure of control over its use.

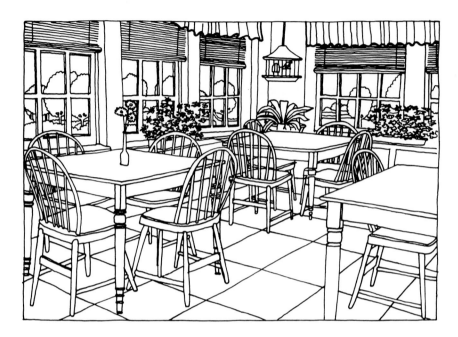

Figure I.3
Wesley Hall, Chelsea, Michigan.

tent possible, the daily schedule was structured around familiar activities of daily living and those familiar settings—living room, den, kitchen—in which such activities occur. The goal of these interventions was the creation of a new form of therapeutic environment for people with dementia who are physically active and well.

> This group does not need the expensive skilled nursing care designed primarily for the physically impaired. Additionally, people with Alzheimer's disease do not require or respond well to the structure and design of the traditional nursing home. They are strongly resistive to the rigid schedules that are often adamantly adhered to . . . by overworked staff. The result is the anger and combativeness attributed to the stereotypical picture of the Alzheimer's victim . . . The findings of the study reported on here give strong evidence of the benefits of the social/residential model in providing therapeutic milieus for persons with dementia (Coons 1987, 9).

This same distinction was clearly drawn by Koncelik (1976) in his proposals for the planning and design of a new form of "open" nursing home. Although not focusing specifically on a dementia population, he argued that the most important quality of such facilities, most often conspicuous by its absence, is that of a sense of "residency." Efforts to provide "homelike" qualities, Koncelik argued, rarely go beyond superficial furnishings and artifacts. A true sense of home, by contrast, is created through opportunities to personalize one's environment and have some measure of control over its use and through both satisfying contacts with others and privacy when that is desired.

Thus, "holding on to home" may be viewed as a superordinate goal in the planning and design of all environments for people with dementia. In addition to working to maintain residents in their own homes as long as possible, it is vitally important that all facilities for people with dementia—day care and respite centers, group homes, assisted living, and long-term care facilities—retain residential qualities to the maximal extent possible.

The Facility Development Process

The design or renovation of facilities for people with dementia—beginning with initial planning and culminating in construction and occupancy—is a complex process. To ensure that every facility realizes its therapeutic potential, it is essential to define carefully those psychological, social, and organizational problems that the resultant building is meant to solve.

Holding On to Home presents a five-stage model of the facility development process: (1) preparation; (2) planning; (3) programing; (4) design, construction, and occupancy; and (5) evaluation. Although these stages partially correspond with the facility development process proposed by the American Institute of Architects (AIA, 1971), the AIA process is clearly weighted toward the "production" aspects of new facilities (i.e., preparation of architectural drawings, bidding, and construction). The goals and contents of *Holding On to Home,* by contrast, are directed more toward the initial phases of problem formulation and design guidance, as well as toward the final phase of systematic evaluation.

The seven chapters of *Holding On to Home* parallel the five stages of this process, with chapters 3 to 5—principles for design—covering the third stage of "programing." Readers can "walk through" the entire process of developing facilities for people with dementia. This process is in no way limited to the planning and design of entire new facilities; it is equally applicable to the renovation of existing settings or individual spaces. It is also hoped that *Holding On to Home* will be of interest to and have value for those who simply wish to learn more about the relationship between the built environment and human behavior.

Preparation

It is essential to understand the needs of people with dementia and the range of environmental options available to them.

This first phase of the facility development process provides the foundation for the phases that follow. Anyone who anticipates involvement in the planning and design of a facility for people with dementia should begin with a clear understanding of the particular environmental needs of this user group as well as of those who serve as caregivers. One must also be aware of the range of environments currently available to people with dementia and of the gaps in this continuum of choices that define the need for new and innovative facility types. Finally, it is essential to appreciate the therapeutic potential of environments for people with dementia and the place of the physical setting within this complex system linking goals, human behavior, and buildings. Thus, chapter 1 provides an introduction to the nature of Alzheimer's disease and presents a set of broadly based therapeutic goals that underlie *Holding On to Home.*

Planning

Typically, it is in the planning stage that basic decisions regarding the functioning of the facility are made. These include formulation of basic organizational goals, structure, and policies, as well as decisions regarding services to be provided, staffing, and number of people to be accommodated. Procedural matters, such as formation of building committees or advisory groups, are also considered at this point. The principles for planning in chapter 2 focus on definition of decisions regarding facility type, community linkages, and staffing.

Programing

A program defines the set of requirements that the architectural design is to satisfy.

The goal of the programing phase is definition of the requirements that the facility to be designed is meant to satisfy. Such requirements may be defined in terms of (1) patterns of behavior to be accommodated in the facility; (2) desired experiential attributes of the environment, such as accessibility or familiarity; and (3) required sensory (e.g., light levels) and spatial (e.g., square footage) properties of individual spaces within the building. Thus, chapters 3 to 5 present principles for design that consider attributes of the environment, relationships between spaces, and requirements for individual activity areas.

Design

This phase results in a complete architectural design for a new facility, typically represented in a combination of drawings and verbal descriptions. Building upon the principles for planning and design, chapter 6 presents a set of "prototypical" designs for innovative facilities serving people with dementia. The nature of each of facility is defined in programmatic terms, including goals, organizational structure and staffing, and population to be served. Drawings for each facility are accompanied by verbal descriptions or "annotations" that describe the designs in greater detail and indicate how key planning and design principles are expressed by them.

Evaluation

Environments for people with dementia may be evaluated in terms of technical, behavioral, and therapeutic concerns.

To complete a cycle of the facility delivery process, the occupied building should be evaluated to assess how well it satisfies the goals specified in the preparation, planning, and programing phases. Such evaluation can include technical issues (are lighting levels in the dining room high enough?), patterns of behavior (is the lounge being used for family visiting?), and experiential and therapeutic concerns (does the lounge provide sufficient stimuli to encourage conversation?). Thus, *Holding On to Home* concludes with a set of questions, paralleling the principles for planning and design, to facilitate evaluation of either existing or proposed environments for people with dementia.

Understanding Costs

One of the most critical questions that arises in any project involving environmental design is related to the "bottom line": How much is it going to cost? It is not possible to give reliable estimates of the exact expenses that will be incurred in the building of a new facility or the renovating of an old one because of the wide variations in labor cost, real estate values, desired materials, state of existing structure (in the case of renovation), scope, and quality of the projects that could be undertaken. However, the following sections sketch briefly the general cost issues that need to be addressed: (1) under "Feasibility Study" we offer an explanation of the factors that determine project feasibility and that are considered when examining the cost of construction in detail; (2) "Project Costs" briefly discusses the three basic types of costs that will be incurred in construction, emphasizing the range and relative proportion of these; and (3) "Process: Decisions and Trade-offs" offers a realistic appraisal of many of the trade-offs and compromises associated with building construction and renovation. For a more extensive review, readers are referred to Rostenberg (1986) and the National Advisory Council on Aging, Government of Canada (1987).

Three preliminary steps must be taken before beginning any building project: (1) establishment of the financial parameters within which the owner and architect will operate; (2) determination of the demands for the services to be provided by the new facility; and (3) investigation of the economic factors that will allow or prevent the success of the venture. These steps require that a preliminary budget be developed and that a market survey and economic feasibility study be undertaken (Table I.1). However, it may be difficult to determine potential demand for innovative services and facilities that do not yet exist or are not widely available in most areas. In these instances, care must be taken to estimate the population that would avail themselves of services or particular facility types, were these available, but who themselves may not have expressed a demand for these services, being unaware of the full range of possible options that might be provided in caring for people with dementia.

Feasibility Study

For any project, three types of cost must always be considered: direct construction costs, indirect costs, and project development costs. At the feasibility stage, these are usually estimated as dollars per square foot. This figure is an average and incorporates the wide cost differences that result from variety in the degree of specialization of individual areas; for example, bathrooms cost more to build than bedrooms because of the expense of the required fixtures and their installation. Table I.2 depicts the three types of costs incurred in the building process and itemizes some of the factors to be considered for each. The estimation of costs is a complex process and will vary according to loca-

Project Costs

Table I.1 *Three Areas That Determine the Feasibility of a Project*

Preliminary Budget	Market Survey	Economic Feasibility
• funds available	• need for service	• funds to develop
• capital required	• community trends	• funds to operate
		• return for your investment

Source: Adapted from Rostenberg 1986.

tion of the facility (both regionally and within specific metropolitan areas). At a later stage, estimation may require the additional services of a cost-estimating consultant.

| Process: Decisions and Trade-offs | Once the decision to build has been made, at least one of the three factors of cost, scope, and quality of construction must remain flexible. For example, should costs escalate unexpectedly during construction, adjustment may have to be made to limit the scope and/or the quality of materials of the structure so that the project can be completed within budget (since the budget or cost of a project is normally inflexible). Of the three factors, construction and programming costs are the least malleable because these are governed by market forces beyond the control of those commissioning the facility. Building is a dynamic process, and planners must be prepared to engage in ongoing decision making on topics as varied as desired materials, present and future spatial requirements, and choice of interior features. Trade-offs are inevitably required.

Kirk, Eichinger, and Spreckelmeyer (1984; in Shumaker & Pequegnat 1989) suggested the following three strategies for improving decision making: multi-objective analysis, life-cycle costing, and postoccupancy evaluation (POE). Through the use of multiobjective analysis, the design option that most clearly matches the stated goals of the building is identified. The process of life-cycle costing compares the advantages and disadvantages of various design alternatives in areas related to building maintenance and operating costs. The final step, POE, assesses the behavior of users in the completed building to determine whether it is meeting their needs and performing the various functions for which it was designed (see chapter 7, "Evaluation of the Environment").

Many of the design principles advanced in *Holding On to Home* specifically address the quality of life of people who reside in long-term care settings. The data presently available suggest that these environmental features may also have a positive effect on residents' behavior in the form of increased or improved function and affect and, as a consequence, may facilitate their care and

Table I.2 *The Three Types of Costs Incurred in Building*

Direct Construction Costs	Indirect Construction Costs	Program Development Costs

• site development
• building costs
• landscaping
• utilities
	• site acquisition
	• contractor's profit and overhead
	• furniture
	• allowances and contingencies
	• miscellaneous costs (e.g., signage)
		• professional fees:
		   architects
		   consultants
		   lawyers
		   accountants
		• site survey
		• insurance
		• postconstruction promotion of service
		• financing
		• permit fees
		• taxes
		• miscellaneous development fees

Source: Adapted from Rostenberg 1986.

encourage family visits (Ohta & Ohta 1988; Lawton, Fulcomer & Kleban 1984). Research in office environments (Brill et al. 1984) indicates that workers are more productive or better satisfied with their employment after changes to their interior environment. While no equally detailed parallel health care studies exist, these findings suggest that the burnout and high turnover rate endemic among staff in long-term care (LTC) units may be ameliorated by improving the environmental quality of these settings.

Brill et al. also pointed out the important fact that construction and building maintenance costs over a twenty- to forty-year building life cycle are only a small part (often as little as 15 percent) of the facility's total costs. The remainder of the total life cycle cost is largely "people-related" (e.g., salaries). Simply put, the operational costs of LTC facilities far outweigh those incurred in constructing the building; a reduction of operational costs through proportionately small present-day investment in enhancing environmental quality may reap substantial future economic benefits through increased staff and resident satisfaction.

Finally, the introduction of positive environmental design features that improve the quality of life need not necessarily represent an added expense. In many instances (e.g., when decisions concerning materials, colors, and internal features are being made), this simply requires the thoughtful application of principles like those presented in *Holding On to Home*.

Overleaf: Hanson Graphic; Stella and Frank Fenner, photographed by Tom Bamberger

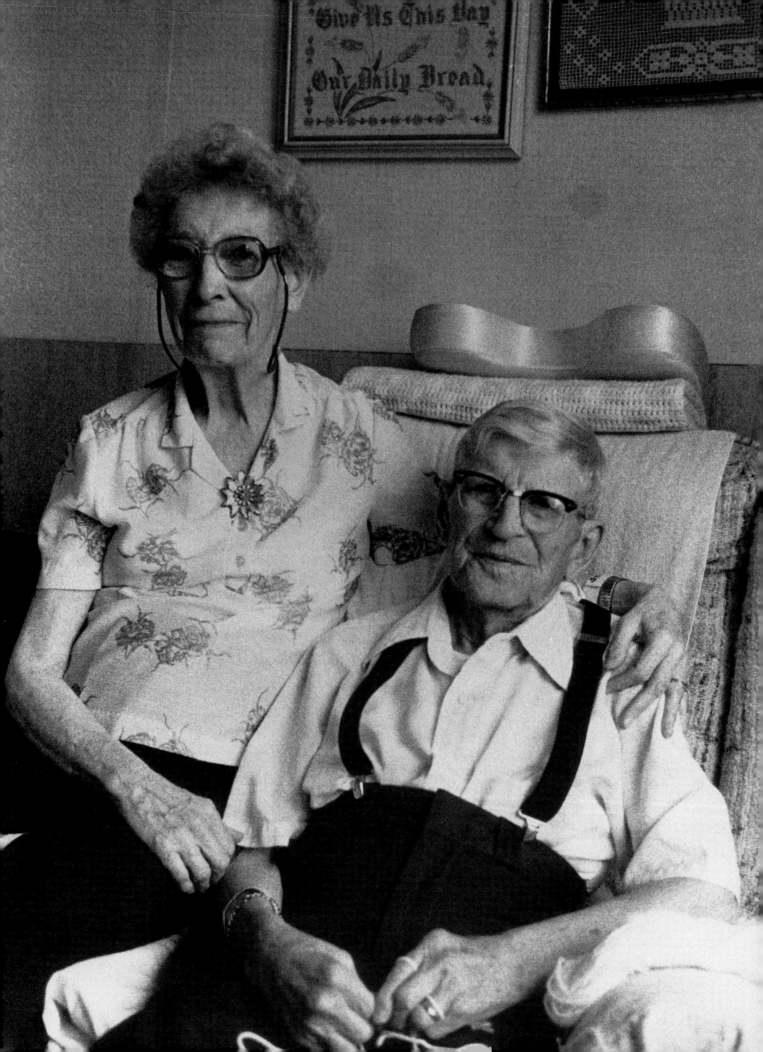

1 *Preparation for Planning and Design*

Although many readers will be familiar with Alzheimer's disease and its characteristics, some may find the following brief review a useful introduction to this topic. The first section, "Basic Facts about Alzheimer's Disease," describes the nature and history of the disease, current research topics, typical symptoms, and their impact. "A Day in The Life" presents two scenarios of typical days in the lives of people with dementia in a vivid portrayal of the real effects of the disease on the victims, their families, and their caregivers. These scenarios are composites of many stories and are representative of the range of circumstances affecting people in this context. The final section introduces a set of nine therapeutic goals, which emerge from the needs of people with dementia and their caregivers. These goals in turn provide broad directions for the "Principles for Planning and Design" that follow in chapters 2 through 5.

The most devastating illness associated with aging is Alzheimer's disease (AD). Known alternately as senile dementia of the Alzheimer's type (SDAT) or dementia of the Alzheimer's type (DAT), this progressive, irreversible neurological disorder is seen in its most severe form in 5 percent of the population over 65 years of age and in 20 percent of the population over 80. Alzheimer's is the most common of the dementing diseases of the elderly, accounting for 50–60 percent of all such cases. In the developed nations, it ranks fourth as a cause of death (after cardiovascular disease, cancer, and cerebrovascular disease).

The severe disabilities resulting from AD, which usually renders its victims helpless, are a major reason for institutionalization and have created a major public health problem. The magnitude of this problem is projected to increase as the number of elderly people in the population increases. In the United States, the number of individuals with severe AD will more than double in the next thirty years (Heston & White 1983; Reisberg 1983; Lindeman 1984; U.S. Congress Office of Technology Assessment 1987).

The first sign of AD is forgetfulness, especially of recent events. Other cognitive functions are gradually compromised: judgment and the ability to orient oneself in space and to time are lost, new learning cannot take place, and expressive speech becomes difficult. Disabling personality changes and mood swings occur. This cognitive, emotional, and behavioral deterioration is not linear and may differ greatly among individuals. Nonetheless, it is relentless, irreversible, and devastating as personal competence is eroded and the afflicted person slips into a state of complete dependence. In the final stages of the disease, which is eventually terminal, neuromuscular changes interfere with mobility and physical abilities (Heston & White 1983; Reisberg 1983; Gilleard 1984; Lindeman 1984; Shamoian 1984; U.S. Congress Office of Technology Assessment 1987). These changes are summarized in Table 1.1.

1.1 Basic Facts about Alzheimer's Disease

- *Dementia is a disease, not a result of normal aging.*

- *Alzheimer's disease usually develops during the person's mid-60s but can occur earlier.*

- *More than 1.5 million U.S. citizens suffer from severe Alzheimer's disease.*

- *Sixty to 70 percent of all patients in nursing homes have Alzheimer's disease.*

Signs and Symptoms

- *Decline in functional, cognitive, emotional, and social abilities.*

- *Reduced mastery and control over the environment.*

- *Prognosis: patients usually die seven to ten years after the onset of dementia, although this period may last up to fifteen to twenty years.*

Table 1.1 *Major Performance Deficits of Alzheimer's Disease*

		Behavioral/Functional	Cognitive	Emotional	Social
Stage 1	**Forgetfulness phase**	Employment: no observable deficits	Difficulty remembering names of people, familiar places and objects	Some anxiety and appropriate concern about symptoms	No observable deficits
	Mild symptoms Diagnosis: Retrospective recognition	Poor performance noted by co-workers	Word-finding deficit that becomes obvious to intimates Possible loss of objects of value	Moderate anxiety about symptoms Irritability	Decreased performance in demanding situations
Stage 2	**Confusional phase**	Difficulty with complex tasks and demanding employment situations	Poor concentration Impairment of reason and judgment Possible episodes of getting lost	Anxiety about symptoms	Inappropriate and embarrassing behavior in social situations
	Moderate symptoms of anger/ guilt, denial, sadness Clear deficits	Inability to perform complex tasks Nocturnal restlessness	Difficulty recalling recent events and aspects of own history Difficulty traveling Financial incompetence Impairment of abstract thought	Denial of symptoms Flat affect Withdrawal from challenging situations	Social ineptitude Social alienation
Stage 3	**Dementia phase**	Inability to initiate or complete purposeful task Nocturnal confusion and wandering	Severe memory loss: inability to recall major aspects of life, names of close family	Denial and shame Catastrophic incidents: irritability, agitation, and violent episodes	Toleration of only simple, structured, familiar social situation Need for reality orientation
	Severe symptoms Separation from self Terminal phase	Incontinence Dependence for all care Loss of basic psychomotor skills (e.g., walking)	Unawareness of time, space, and events Loss of speech Abulia (loss of intentionality) Inability to recall own name	Personality changes: paranoia, hallucinations, delusions Obsessional behavior	No social interaction

Etiology

- *Diagnosis is difficult.*
- *Cause is unknown.*
- *AD develops regardless of gender, race, or social status.*

The etiology, or cause, of Alzheimer's disease is unknown. Early signs and symptoms may be mistaken for normal aging and, as the disease progresses, are difficult to distinguish from those of other dementias. Therefore, the goal of diagnosis is to rule out other forms of irreversible dementias, as well as reversible dementias, which may respond to treatment. A medical history, a physical examination, psychological and laboratory tests, and various kinds of brain scans are usually necessary (Heston & White 1983; Gubrium 1986; U.S. Congress Office of Technology Assessment 1987). Drugs are sometimes used to ameliorate symptoms such as agitation and paranoia, but there is currently no treatment that can arrest the underlying pathological condition of AD.

The major performance deficits of Alzheimer's disease can be divided into four categories: behavioral/functional, cognitive, emotional, and social. Behavioral/functional deficits include those changes associated with dementia that result in impaired task performance (e.g., reduced ability to deal with demanding employment situations) and significant physical changes (e.g., incontinence). Cognitive deficits are those changes that result in difficulty in mental functioning (e.g., remembering names, abstract thinking). Emotional deficits include changes in affective response (e.g., personality changes and catastrophic reactions).

In Table 1.1, these four types of performance deficits are shown with the stages of the disease (as described by Reisberg 1983) in which they are likely to occur. Stage 1 is the period in which symptoms are first likely to be noticed; there may be anxiety and some decrease in task performance and social aptitude, but there is not typically a diagnosis of Alzheimer's disease at this stage. In stage 2 there are increased deficits, including major changes in the ability to perform tasks, to concentrate, to remember recent events, and to conduct reasonable or abstract thought. There are also significant decreases in the display of emotion and in the ability to function in social situations. Stage 3 is the final stage, in which the major identifiable characteristics of dementia are likely to surface, including wandering, incontinence, severe loss of memory and orientation, severe and significant changes in personality, and an inability to tolerate most social situations.

Most people with dementia are cared for at home, at least in the earlier stages of the disease (U.S. Congress Office of Technology Assessment 1987). The unrelenting demands placed upon the caregiver, usually the spouse or a close family member, create what Mace and Rabins (1981) characterized as the "36-hour day." Without respite, the caregiver often becomes the second victim of the disease.

The following symptoms are identified by caregivers as most problematic (Pynoos & Ohta 1988):

Cognitive symptoms:

- extreme memory failure
- inability to communicate
- disorientation to time and place

Functional symptoms:

difficulties with activities of daily living, including

- bathing
- dressing
- eating
- handling money
- cooking
- cleaning house

The Effect on Caregivers

"I was out of energy, out of patience . . . and I was afraid I was out of love, because I was starting to scream at him . . . and he hit me one time. Every day he is slowly dying and part of me is dying with him, and our marriage is dying with him . . . I am not widowed, not married . . . what am I?" (Wife-caregiver) (Gnaedinger 1989)

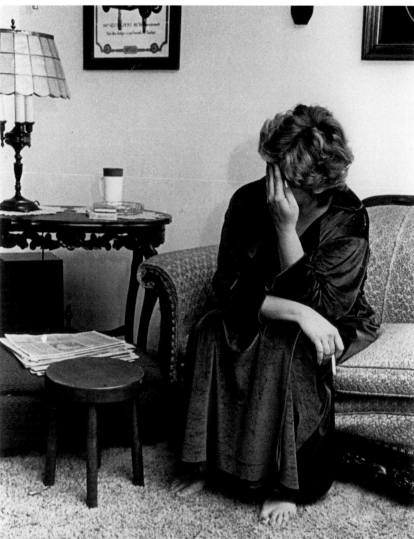

Pat Schmidt, photographed by Robert Glick

- taking medication
- incontinence
- night walking and wandering

Emotional symptoms:

- restlessness
- demanding, critical, accusatory, and volatile behavior
- violence to self and others
- withdrawal

Stress experienced by caregivers has been the focus of a number of studies (Rabins 1982; Gilleard 1984; Kelly 1984; Pynoos & Ohta 1988). These researchers generally agree on the issues that are seen as the most difficult for caregivers to handle. However, there is variability in the characteristics of individuals with dementia. Symptoms that cause problems with care are primarily associated with the later stages of AD and include difficulties with activities of daily living (ADL), getting lost, unsafe behavior, constant wandering and rummaging, disorientation in time and space, agitation, occasional violent or catastrophic behavior, and, conversely, withdrawal. Eventually, the person suffering from Alzheimer's disease cannot be left alone, and the caregiver ultimately becomes bound to the home almost completely. Supervision and care are required at all times (Kelly 1984; U.S. Congress Office of Technology Assessment 1987).

Support for caregivers includes providing information about the disease, auxiliary care relief services, and assistance with planning for the advanced stages of the disease. In particular, families need to seek legal advice regarding issues of ownership and the transfer of financial responsibilities. They may also need help with choosing appropriate institutional care, should that be deemed necessary (Heston & White 1983; Kelly 1984; Lindeman 1984; U.S. Congress Office of Technology Assessment 1987).

Supportive therapies that help both the victim and the family adjust to the progressive decline by improving coping and daily living skills constitute the main assistance that can be offered. Activities and environmental modifications that help to minimize dysfunction and maximize remaining capabilities should also be implemented. In particular, it is important to prevent the development of secondary physical and psychiatric health problems.

Ensuring safety is a concern throughout the course of the disease. The overriding goal, however, should be the preservation of the individual's comfort and dignity. This is aided by allowing control over the environment and over daily living activities whenever reasonable and possible (Heston & White 1983; Reisberg 1983; Gilleard 1984; Lindeman 1984; Shamoian 1984; U.S. Congress Office of Technology Assessment 1987).

Intervention:

- *Deal with paradoxical behaviors.*

- *Help families deal with their new roles and sense of despair.*

- *Help people with dementia deal with the frustrations of diminishing memory and skills.*

- *Help prevent accidents and wandering away from home.*

- *Stress the significance of comfort, control, and dignity.*

The Environmental Context of Dementia

Despite popular stereotypes, not all people with dementia reside in nursing homes. While they are overrepresented in long-term care facilities, up to three times as many people with dementia reside in the community (Pynoos & Ohta 1988). The range of environmental options is presently quite limited, offering essentially four choices to people with dementia and their caregivers (Cohen et al. 1988).

People with dementia most often reside at home (fig. 1.1); in most cases, this is also the environment of preference for as long as possible. As the disease progresses, however, stress upon the caregiver and the inability to care properly for the person with dementia at home may necessitate the choice of an alternate setting.

In response to increasing demands on caregivers at home, day care facilities (fig. 1.2) provide an alternative environment for people with dementia for periods of a few hours to a full day. At this point in the development of day care facilities, there seem to be few consistent patterns in their size, architectural character, or location in the community.

Group homes are another existing option, although they are relatively limited in number at present. These are most often existing houses within the community that have been modified to accommodate a small group of residents and one or two caregivers. Group size varies from state to state but is typically eight or more (fig. 1.3). Architectural intervention takes the form of

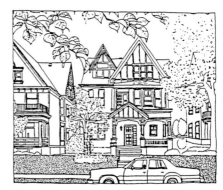

Figure 1.1
Most people with dementia live in single family homes.

Figure 1.2
Typically, day care centers are housed in an existing facility, such as a community center or church basement. This floor plan illustrates a common arrangement.

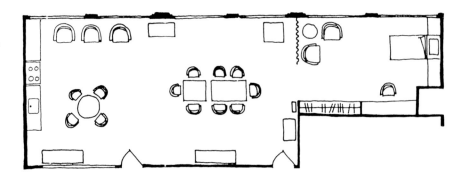

space expansion to accommodate all residents, response to life safety require-ments (such as the installation of sprinklers), and the creation of protected outdoor space.

Finally, long-term care facilities (fig. 1.4) are the only environmental op-tion available to many people with dementia no longer able to live at home, even with assistance. Increasing numbers of nursing homes now offer "special care units" for people with Alzheimer's disease. However, the therapeutic in-tentions, as well as the organizational and architectural structure of such units, vary widely (Ohta & Ohta 1988; Mathew et al. 1988).

There is a far from perfect correlation between facility type and level of impairment of people with dementia. Those cared for at home often have symptoms as severe as dementia patients in long-term care facilities (Lowen-thal, Berkman and associates 1967).

Many of the problems experienced by people with dementia and their care-givers are linked directly to the planning and design of the environment. Among a sample of caregivers studied by Pynoos and Ohta (1988), four of the

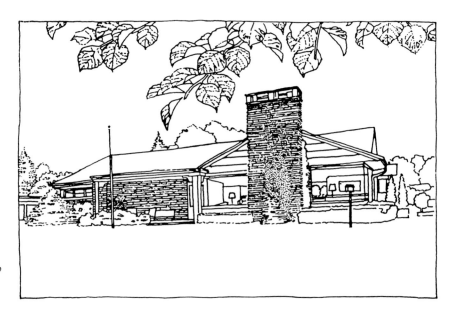

Figure 1.3
The number of residents in a group home is influenced by state regulation, but a small group (six to eight) is likely to be perceived as most homelike and familiar.

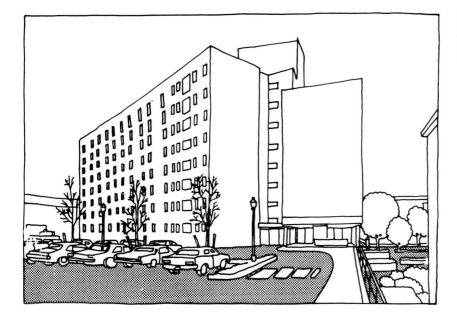

Figure 1.4
Long-term care facilities can appear imposing and institutional and are not usually characterized as homelike or residential.

ten most frequent problems focused on activities of daily living (dressing, preparing meals, bathing, and house cleaning), which may be either facilitated or hindered by the design of equipment, furnishings, or spaces. Of the ten problems that elicited extreme negative reactions from caregivers, four dealt with issues of wandering and spatial orientation; research suggests that effective spatial orientation is clearly linked to the organization of the architectural environment (Weisman 1987). More generally, the presence or absence of a given facility type (e.g., respite care) within a community may influence the health and well-being of both people with dementia and their caregivers.

1.2 A Day in the Life

Jerry Schmidt

At 5:15 in the morning, Pat Schmidt is awakened by the sound of her husband fumbling downstairs in the kitchen. Though weary, she is quickly out of bed to check on Jerry. Walking into the kitchen, Pat sees Jerry standing at the window, intently peering outside. The dog is barking to go out, but he doesn't seem to notice. Jerry used to wait here for his friend Joe to pick him up for work; Pat thinks that may be what Jerry is doing now. She gently reminds Jerry that he retired three years ago and asks him if he wants to go back to sleep.

Jerry is only forty-five years old; however, he had to retire at age forty-two, after he was diagnosed as having Alzheimer's disease. It is unusual for Alzheimer's disease to occur in so young a person; however, the symptoms are the same (and equally devastating) at any age. For the preceding twenty years, Jerry had been a hardworking general laborer at a nearby meat packing plant; he had always been a lover of the outdoors and a family person. He and Pat had spent much of their free time with their large family, making plans for the things they would do together when the children grew up. This dream, however, seems to have fallen apart.

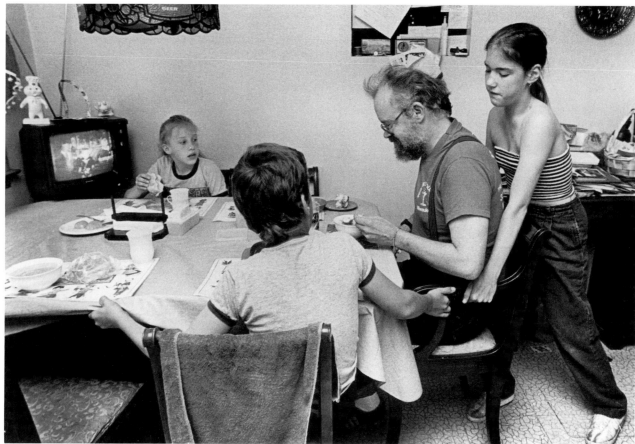

Jerry Schmidt and family, photographed by Robert Glick

At first, Jerry's symptoms of forgetfulness seemed to be little more than absentmindedness. He was unable to remember the names of places they often visited, would return from the store having forgotten what he meant to get, and would miss activities or appointments that he had scheduled. Pat began to compensate for his forgetfulness by reminding him of the names of people they would see at a neighborhood party and excusing his forgetfulness to friends by telling them that things were especially stressful at work lately. Pat would spell out directions to destinations in advance, pretending to make conversation: "Why don't we drive along the beach and take a right at First Street to get to your sister's?" She would volunteer to accompany Jerry when he took a walk in the evening, afraid that he would not be able to find his way back alone.

It soon became apparent that something serious was wrong. Jerry became easily confused and did not always make sense when he spoke, often repeating himself several times or interrupting a conversation with completely unrelated comments. He lost interest in his hobbies, giving up bowling and hunting. He spent virtually no time in his workshop or, when there, merely sat passively. Sometimes, Jerry would get angry for no apparent reason—lashing out at Pat or their children over insignificant incidents or nothing at all. Most of the time, however, he just sat in his chair, listless and uninterested or unaware of the activity around him. Gradually, he became more and more careless about his grooming and required assistance in bathing and dressing.

Having taken Jerry upstairs, Pat helps him to wash and get dressed. It is important for her, and for Jerry, to keep him as independent and autonomous as possible. Pat has labeled the locations of his clothes and toiletries and lets him make as many decisions for himself as he can handle. She has posted reminders and instructions (such as "change your clothes") for Jerry, but she finds that she has to double-check after him, turning off the tap when he leaves the water running and unplugging appliances that he plugs in and then forgets to use. She has had grab bars installed in the bathroom and a second hand rail installed along the stairs, and she hopes that these devices will ex-

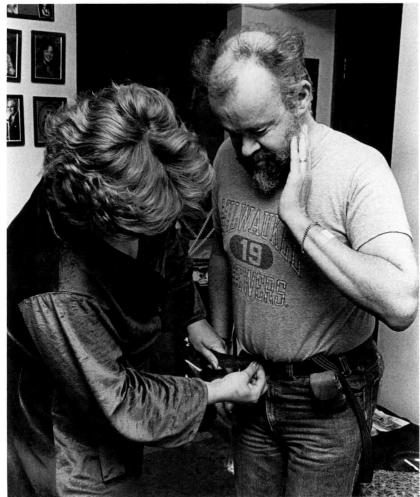

Pat and Jerry Schmidt, photographed by Robert Glick

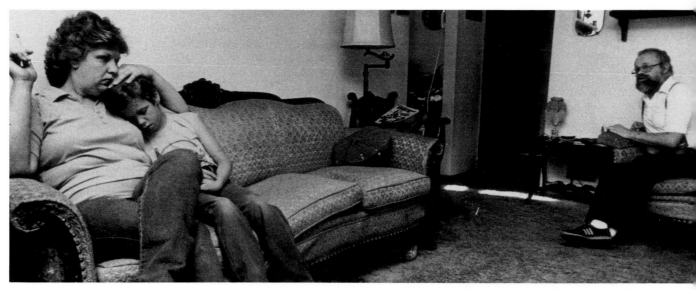

Jerry Schmidt and family, photographed by Susie Post

tend the time that Jerry is able to get around on his own. With the help of the kids, Pat pushed all the living room furniture against the walls to clear a path for Jerry's endless wandering throughout the house. She worries, however, that if she makes too many changes Jerry will become disoriented and confused.

Later that day, during breakfast, Pat's mother stops to visit. Pat's parents live right next door to Pat's family, which has been a great source of support and assistance for Pat. Worries and demands associated with Jerry's illness have become a constant topic of conversation between Pat and her mother. Again this morning, Pat expresses concern about managing the house and family by herself but doesn't feel that she could afford to hire someone to help with the cleaning and maintenance.

Pat's parents do everything they can to help their daughter and her family, including helping to keep an eye on Jerry or the kids so that Pat can get out of the house to run errands or to attend the Alzheimer's support group that she supervises once every month. It would be very difficult for Pat to leave Jerry with strangers, so she feels lucky that her parents live close enough to be so much help. She is also proud of the way that the kids have pitched in to help out with their father. It is difficult for them to understand what is happening to Jerry, and Pat tries to explain things in a way that will not frighten them.

Luckily for both Pat and Jerry, there is a local day care center that Jerry can attend a couple of times a week; the day care center even sends a van to pick him up and bring him home. Pat is sure that the socializing and activities at the day care center help to jog Jerry's memory and keep him involved with other people; she's relieved that he seems to enjoy himself there, even though he usually just sits and watches most of the activities.

Jerry's illness has been tough on Pat and their children, but Pat hopes that, with the help of the local day care center, the Alzheimer's support group, and her parents, she will be able to continue to take care of Jerry at home for a

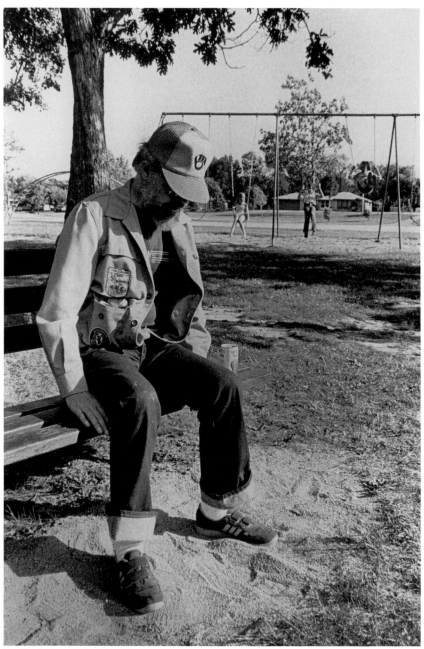

Jerry Schmidt, photographed by Robert Glick

while yet. Eventually, however, she realizes that they will probably have to place Jerry in a nursing home. Pat tries to stay optimistic and upbeat, but sometimes she can't help becoming overwhelmed by what is slowly happening to her husband. There seems to be so little that she can do to help him.

Janice Hollander

Even though it is still dark outside, the lights in room 107 are switched on, and the nurse wakes Janice up. Because of the schedule in the nursing home and the number of residents, Janice must now get up at 6:30 a.m., despite the fact that she has always been accustomed to sleeping later. Paula, the nurse, helps Janice to the bathroom to wash and dress, handing her the clothes she is to put on. Janice often rummages through her own and others' possessions, throwing things around or taking out articles of clothing and hiding them or carrying them to other parts of the unit, where she forgets and leaves them. The nurses now find it easier simply to keep Janice's clothes locked up and to provide one dress at a time. Once again, however, Janice's slippers are missing, probably taken by another resident. After Janice is dressed, Paula leads her back to a chair in her room and promises to come back to take her to breakfast. Janice sits, occasionally dozing off, and waits for someone to return.

Janice Hollander is a 79-year-old widow. Although still mobile, she has Alzheimer's disease; for the past six months, she has been a resident at Lakeview Home for the Aged. A high school social science teacher and then a principal, Janice lost her husband less than a year after her retirement. She continued to live alone for seven years but, after being diagnosed as having Alzheimer's disease, she moved in with her son Tom and his family. During the past year, as concern for Janice's safety and the stress on Tom's family both increased, it was decided to move her to Lakeview.

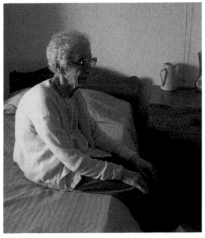

Anna Pappas, at Marina View Manor, HCR Inc., Milwaukee, Wis.; photographed by Tom Bamberger

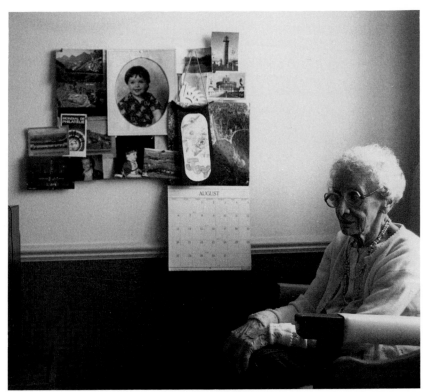

Anna Pappas, at Marina View Manor, HCR Inc., Milwaukee, Wis.; photographed by Tom Bamberger

After a twenty-minute wait, a nurse's aide comes to take Janice to breakfast. Janice is confused because she does not recognize or remember the aide; however, the woman is friendly and patient and convinces Janice to come to the dining room. As they leave her room, they hear a commotion in the corridor; a buzzer is ringing at the nurse's station, and an aide is running to an emergency exit at the far end of the hall. A resident of the Alzheimer's unit has opened the fire door, and the magnetic tape attached to his ankle has activated the alarm. Janice becomes agitated because of all the commotion; this is a relatively common occurrence on the unit as wanderers approach the exit at the termination of the dead-end corridor.

Breakfast trays are already on the tables when Janice gets to the dining room, and she sits at her usual place. As always, there is more food on the tray than Janice is accustomed to eating for breakfast, and she is not yet hungry this early in the morning. During breakfast, Paula and the other nurses try to encourage interaction by grouping residents with others at the same level of cognitive ability. Some patients must be fed by staff, and others use their fingers to eat, but Janice is still able to feed herself reasonably well.

After breakfast, Janice remains in the dining room for art therapy. The activity director tells the group that they are going to paint pictures that they will be able to put up in the hallway. Most of the residents, unable to do much on their own, require a great deal of staff assistance. Others in the room do not participate at all. Some restlessly wander the corridors, stopping at the nurse's station to ask questions; others watch television in the day room, and some simply sleep in their rooms. Janice works on her painting for a while but then forgets what she is doing and remains sitting, watching the others, for the rest of the hour.

Janice's son Tom makes his weekly visit during his lunch hour. Although Janice does not always recognize who he is, his presence almost always brings a faint smile to her face.

Tom tries to get his mother interested in the painting project again but gives up and goes to speak with the program director about Janice's condition. Remembering what a bright, energetic woman Janice had been, Tom now finds it difficult to see her so helpless and disinterested. She had always been an excellent cook and had loved to spend time in the kitchen or puttering about the house. Now, she seems to have no interest in most activities provided at Lakeview. Tom still feels guilty that his family is no longer able to care for Janice at home, but someone must be with her at all times. Because she can no longer climb stairs, their house would have required either a chair lift or a new first floor bedroom and bath. Also, she was beginning to lose continence, and this was a problem with which the entire family found it hard to cope.

Tom hands Janice a picture that his young daughter, Jennifer, drew at school. Jennifer refuses to come to the nursing home; she no longer recognizes this frail woman as the grandmother she used to know.

By the time Tom must leave to return to work, his mother has had lunch and is asleep in her room. Not wanting to disturb her, he gently tacks Jennifer's picture to the corkboard beside Janice's bed. Walking toward the lobby, his mind races with emotions and concerns, but most of all he is grateful to the

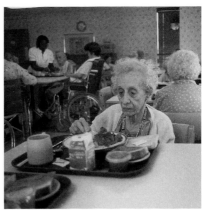

Anna Pappas, at Marina View Manor, HCR Inc., Milwaukee, Wis.; photographed by Tom Bamberger

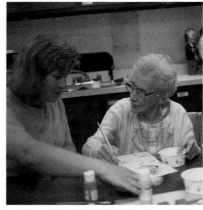

Anna Pappas and Krista Elich, at Marina View Manor, HCR Inc., Milwaukee, Wis.; photographed by Tom Bamberger

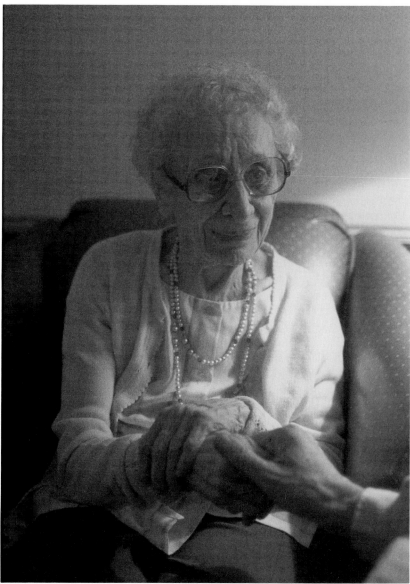

Anna Pappas, at Marina View Manor, HCR Inc., Milwaukee, Wis.; photographed by Tom Bamberger

people who take care of Janice. He appreciates the nurses and caregivers who seem concerned about her in spite of the busy pace and the large number of other residents on the unit. He goes back to work, wondering whether the decision to move Janice to Lakeview had been the best one but knowing that he had few other alternatives.

1.3 Therapeutic Goals

As illustrated in the profiles of Jerry Schmidt and Janice Hollander, the environments occupied by people with dementia may have significant consequences—either positive or negative—for the quality of their lives. The neighborhood in which Jerry and Pat reside offers a senior center, transportation, and other familiar resources. At the same time, Pat recognizes that it will become increasingly difficult for Jerry to remain in their current home and that alternative places of residence are limited and may be less able to provide Jerry with the levels of activity, familiarity, and support that she feels he requires.

Similarly, Tom Hollander's decision to relocate his mother to a long-term care facility was the result of the limitations of his current home, which left Janice isolated on the second floor and imposed severe caregiving burdens on his family. While Janice's needs for safety and security are now met, Tom worries that her remaining capabilities are not exercised to the greatest extent possible in her new living environment.

Concern with goals such as safety, security, familiarity, and social contact figure prominently in the literature on environments for people with dementia (Rand et al. 1987). Particularly useful treatments are provided by Calkins (1987, 1988) and Lawton (1987). Calkins defined a set of "environment and behavior issues," such as wayfinding, privacy and socialization, safety and security, and activities of daily living, which can be viewed as goals for a treatment environment for people with dementia. Lawton presented goals applicable to the full range of person-environment interactions, including such settings for people with dementia as home and institution and both new and existing facilities. While one clearly cannot make specific planning or design decisions on the basis of broad statements regarding "preservation of dignity" or "maximizing of independence," such goals serve to highlight desired relationships between people with dementia and the environments they occupy and to provide direction for policy, programing, and design decisions.

Goal statements serve to highlight desired relationships between people with dementia and the environments they occupy.

To establish a basis for the principles for planning and design presented in chapters 2 through 5, the following nine therapeutic goals have been synthesized from the literature. This set of goals is, of course, an abstraction; in some instances goals may overlap or even conflict with one another. Nevertheless, an understanding of such goals can sensitize the reader to some of the higher level imperatives to which any environment for people with dementia should respond. Furthermore, it is often through efforts to accommodate therapeutic goals that are inherently and necessarily in conflict that the richest and most creative strategies for problem solving emerge (Alexander 1969).

It is often through efforts to reconcile goals that are seemingly in conflict that the most creative solutions emerge.

To the extent possible, each of the following therapeutic goals is illustrated in terms of both architectural design and policy/program implications. In this way designers may gain a better sense of the organizational context within which they operate, while caregivers can better understand and appreciate the potential role of the physical environment as a medium for therapeutic intervention. These mutually reinforcing perspectives will assist in the creation of integrated social, organizational, and physical environments.

Ensuring that users sustain no harm is the first imperative of any therapeutic environment. As emphasized by Calkins (1988), people with dementia are potentially vulnerable as a consequence of cognitive impairment and of physical disabilities related to the process of aging and to the progress of the disease. Thus, it is essential to ensure the physical safety and psychological security of people with dementia.

Although concerns of safety and security are most often reflected in codes and standards, very few such regulatory documents have yet been promulgated specifically for environments for people with dementia. Furthermore, existing codes deal with relatively few of the physical and organizational features of

Goal 1: Ensure Safety and Security

As a consequence of both physical and cognitive impairments, people with dementia are potentially more vulnerable to environmental effects.

these environments. With respect to the physical setting, such regulations most often deal with basic life safety issues (e.g., fire retardant construction, provision of an adequate number of emergency exits). On the organizational side, requirements regarding staff training and staffing ratios are likewise directed toward ensuring the safety and security of people with dementia. This goal must be balanced against other equally important therapeutic goals—for example, provision of opportunities for autonomy and control for people with dementia.

Other ways in which the physical environment might affect the safety and security of people with dementia are less obvious and probably less often considered in requirements for planning and design. These include potential hazards that might emerge during normal use of a facility (e.g., absence of grab bars or an unsecured gas range). On a larger scale, some floor plans might be more effective than others in facilitating staff supervision and surveillance of a special care unit.

Goal 2: Support Functional Ability through Meaningful Activity

Engaging in meaningful activities can help to maintain competence and enhance self-esteem.

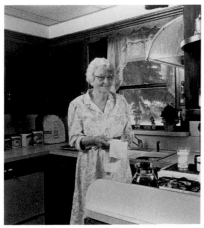

Photo courtesy of Carolyn Lookabill, HCR, Inc.

Both Mace (1987) and Peppard (1986) emphasized the importance of maintaining those abilities not totally impaired by dementia. Support of the highest level of functional ability, as in performance of the activities of daily living or through meaningful activity programs, can have important and positive implications for the sense of competence and self-esteem of people with dementia. Coons (1987) emphasized the need for availability of normal social roles for people with dementia rather than that of a "frail, sick patient." Some positive and useful roles include friend, citizen, consumer, worker, and user of leisure time. Involvement in activities that encourage assumption of some of these roles represents a way to maintain the highest level of functional capabilities for people with dementia. Staff can reinforce this further by allowing people with dementia to carry out those activities of daily living of which they are still capable, even if this takes additional time. It is all too easy to lose patience and quickly perform these tasks for impaired persons rather than allow them to care for themselves. This is reflected in the phenomenon of excess disability "in which the level of function is poorer than the patient's physiological capability" (Kahn 1975), leading to a focus on inherent helplessness rather than support in areas of functioning that remain reasonably intact.

As with safety and security, the maintenance of functional abilities and the performance of the activities of daily living may be negatively influenced by both physical and cognitive impairments. Similarly, the full range of potential caregivers—family, friends, and facility staff—can help people with dementia to maintain and maximize their level of functioning. As further described in goal 4, they should be allowed and encouraged to do everything of which they are capable without being, or feeling, overly taxed by the demands of a task. Prosthetic devices in the physical setting can compensate for some disease related losses; to the extent that such physical supports are employed and effective, the time and energies of caregivers are freed for other tasks.

Dementia may engender confusion and disorientation with respect to time and place. Program, policy, and design should all work to maximize the awareness and orientation of people with dementia to their physical and social environment, assisting them in "knowing where they are" in terms of time, place, and social situation so that they naturally engage in appropriate behaviors. A regular daily program of activities, featuring well-established "temporal landmarks" such as meals, can provide both structure and predictability (Heston & White 1983). This does not necessarily imply "reality therapy" in the traditional sense; indeed, Coons and Spencer (1983) suggested that "reality orientation is seen only as a natural outgrowth of the person's involvement in a complex and purposeful environment."

Maximizing environmental awareness and orientation of people with dementia also requires response to problems of wandering. For some individuals, wandering is a natural response and an outlet for energy; however, people should not be forced to wander as the result of disorientation brought on by a confusing, illegible, unpredictable environment. Therapeutic environments should assist people with dementia in identifying their present location and in following clear paths to desired destinations.

Goal 3: Maximize Awareness and Orientation

Both setting and program should be clearly structured to provide architectural and temporal landmarks.

As a consequence of age and disease-related decrements in sensory and cognitive processes, attention must be given to the intensity and patterning of sensory and social stimulation presented to people with dementia. They may not be able to process high levels of stimulation without experiencing overload and distress; conversely, many institutional settings represent a degree of sensory and social deprivation that is clearly not therapeutic and that exacerbates dementia-related symptoms (Lawton 1981). It is essential to provide regulated stimulation and appropriate challenge. In Mace's terms, the goal is one of "stimulation but not stress" (1987).

The physical setting can contribute to the moderation of stimulation and challenge through provision of private spaces for reflection and retreat (Calkins 1986) as well as moderation of sensory input—especially visual and auditory input (Pastalan 1979; Koncelik 1979). Some degree of structure and consistency in daily patterns of living can further serve to moderate stimulation and create a relaxing and comfortable environment for people with dementia. It should be borne in mind, however, that rigid routines and inflexible schedules are nontherapeutic and even stress producing (Coons 1987). Consistent with this approach, the "progressively lowered stress threshold" model (Hall & Buckwalter 1986) monitors, modifies, and simplifies activities and environmental stimuli to minimize anxious behaviors resulting from overload. The goal is spontaneity in daily activities within a defined routine, which does not require unattainable challenges for people with dementia.

Goal 4: Provide Opportunities for Stimulation and Change

Sensory and social stimulation should be carefully regulated to avoid either deprivation or overload.

The world of people with dementia shrinks greatly, with maximal control limited to that which can be seen and touched. Regulation of stimulation and challenge (goal 4) and a focus on the healthy and familiar (goal 7) may both

Goal 5: Maximize Autonomy and Control

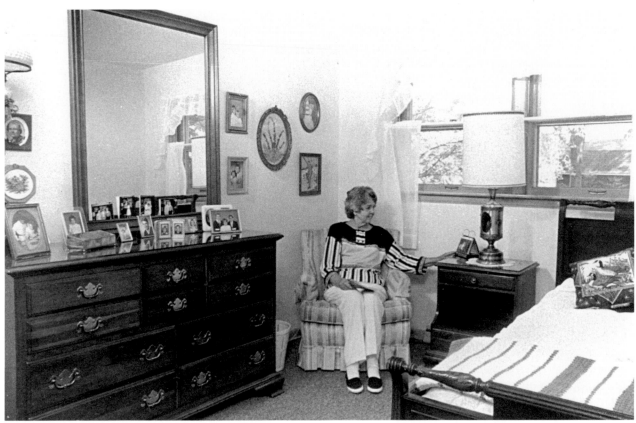

Photo courtesy of Carolyn Lookabill, HCR, Inc.

To the extent possible, people with dementia should be encouraged to make decisions regarding their own environment.

be facilitated if people with dementia have opportunities for some degree of autonomy and control. Often, dependency in long-term care facilities is fostered by environmental factors and specific learned interactions ("learned helplessness"), as well as by biological deterioration (Hofland 1988). Both physical design and organizational policy can support "personalization" of the living environment; for residents of group homes or long-term care facilities, this may include bringing along valued furniture or artifacts from one's home or having some choice in selection of bedspread or drapes. Finally, as Coons and Spencer (1983) suggested, people with dementia should, to the greatest extent possible, have the ability to make decisions and to take responsibility for their own lives. This can be supported by limiting staff assistance to clinical requirements and encouraging maintenance of functional abilities and independence of residents (Hofland 1988).

Dementing diseases exhibit great variation, both across people and within individuals over even relatively short periods. Alzheimer's disease units typically must contend with both turnover in resident population and aging of this same population as they progress through the disease. Thus, it is essential to respond to changing needs and capabilities of people with dementia. Facilities must determine the range of ability or disability and the degree of integration or segregation of groups, at varying stages of the disease, that they wish to accommodate. However, even in integrated settings, segregation does tend to occur in terms of floors occupied, location of bedrooms, sitting spaces regularly occupied, and dining areas; interactions may also occur within, rather than across, groups (Harris, Lipman & Slater 1977).

Goal 6: Adapt to Changing Needs

Dementias exhibit great variation across people and within people over time.

People with dementia are confronted with an ongoing series of changes both in themselves and in their world. It is important, to the extent possible, to maintain ties to that which is healthy, familiar, and comfortable. Coons and Spencer (1983) advocated a therapeutic milieu intentionally patterned after the outside community, with an emphasis on wellness and opportunities for residents to integrate experiences and relationships with their past lives. The creation of a healthy and familiar therapeutic environment also provides the sort of "soft transition" from community to institution suggested by Mace and Rabins (1981) and contributes to more positive feelings on the part of the families of people with dementia. In addition to organizational and architectural means, links to the past can also be maintained by visitation of family and friends. This is probably the predominant mode by which residents have contact with the world outside, providing both positive therapeutic benefits and personal services for residents.

Goal 7: Establish Links to the Healthy and Familiar

Environments for people with dementia should maintain as many links as possible with their past lives.

The need for socialization is a fundamental need for human beings. Communication, both verbal and nonverbal, forms the essence of human socialization. Because the progression of dementing illness is typically associated with a gradual decline in communication functions, resulting in social isolation and depressed cognitive functioning for patients, it is important that facilities provide opportunities for social contact among people with dementia; maintenance of communication and interaction provides continued stimulation and exercise of higher cognitive processes, such as thinking and memory. While environments are not deterministic in promoting social contact, some support socialization more than others; this potential has been characterized by Lawton (1987) as the "social affordance" of a setting. Even the simple manipulation of putting chairs around a table rather than against a wall or in an elliptical arrangement may increase social contact (Peterson et al. 1977). On a larger architectural scale, the Weiss Institute of the Philadelphia Geriatric Center demonstrated that physical interventions can assist in promoting social interaction among dementia patients (Liebowitz, Lawton & Waldman

Goal 8: Provide Opportunities for Socialization

Continuing social contact is a significant therapeutic activity.

33

1979). Thus, environments for people with dementia can and should encourage socialization among residents by creating opportunities for communication through physical design, program, and policy.

Goal 9: Protect the Need for Privacy

People with dementia should have access to a range of public and private activities and spaces.

As a consequence of the need for surveillance and assistance with activities of daily living, relocation to an institutional setting often results in an accompanying loss of privacy for people with dementia. It is often both expensive and difficult to provide physical privacy, but environments for people with dementia should allow residents choices between solitude and participation in activities by providing a range of public to private spaces. Clearly defined boundaries between public and private spaces ensure that there is no ambiguity between that which is shared and that which belongs to an individual. Demarcation of territorial boundaries in the bedrooms of institutionalized elderly can result in an increase in self-satisfaction and mental status among both organically impaired and unimpaired residents (Nelson & Paluck 1980). Organizational policies such as training staff to knock before entering rooms can support individual's need for and right to privacy.

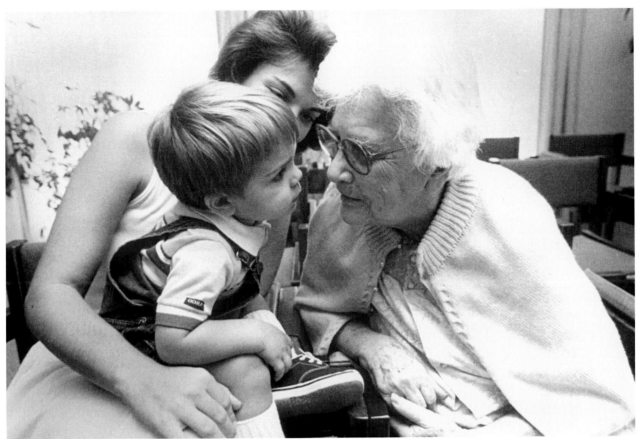

Photo courtesy of Carolyn Lookabill, HCR, Inc.

Overleaf: Hanson Graphic; photograph courtesy of American Medical Services, Inc.; photographed by Walter Sheffer and Sue Bartfield

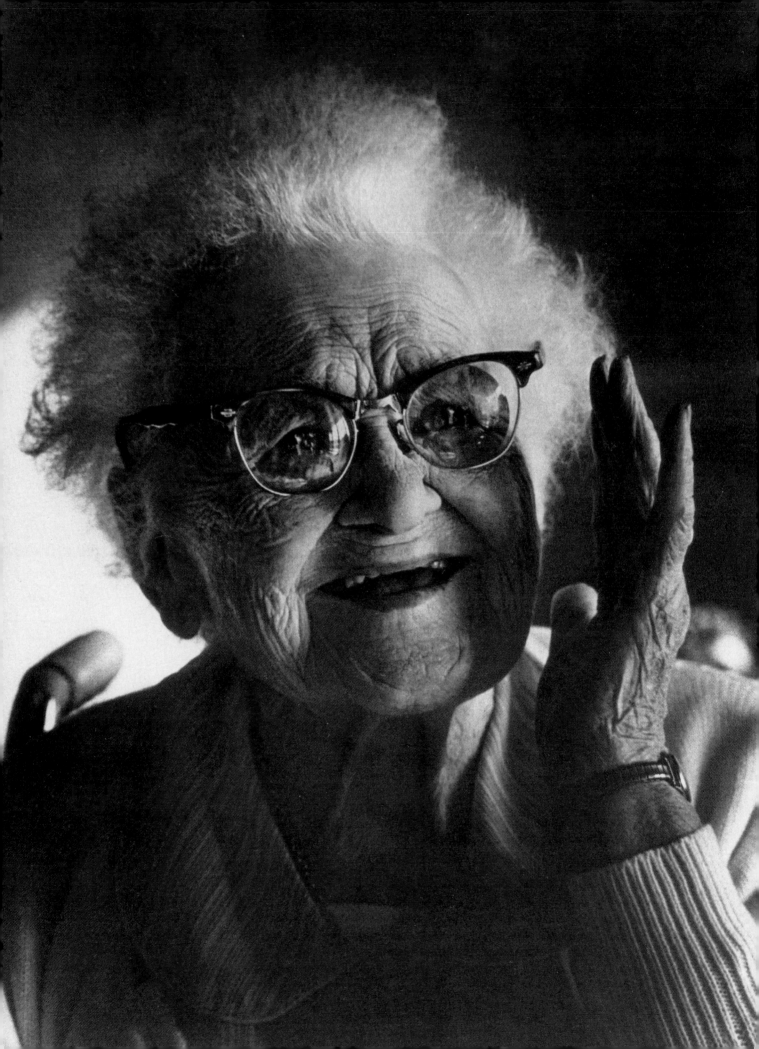

2 *Principles for Planning*

This first set of three principles deals with broad-based planning decisions: (1) where along the continuum of care a given facility should fall; (2) to what extent services must be provided on site, as opposed to being provided in the community; and (3) how many people shall compose a "group" for treatment and/or housing.

These principles, like those to follow in chapters 3, 4, and 5, have a consistent structure. Reflecting the nature of the environment as a complex system, each principle is presented in three parts: (1) needs of people with dementia and their caregivers as well as the therapeutic goals that emerge from these needs; (2) policy, planning, and design concepts that respond to and reconcile multiple therapeutic goals; and (3) illustrations of one or more ways in which these concepts can be effectively implemented.

Thus, each principle begins with "behavioral" concerns of people and organizations and concludes with environmental decision making. It is hoped that this three-part structure will assist planners and designers in understanding and appreciating the social/psychological dimensions that underlie their decisions; conversely, health and social service providers may more clearly recognize the role of the physical setting as a potential therapeutic resource in their work.

2.1 Responsive Continuum of Care

Environmental options available to people with dementia can be seen as a continuum from continued residence at home to day care, group homes, and traditional long-term care environments. The development of additional options along this continuum is both possible and desirable. A more responsive continuum of care can provide a broader range of services for people at all stages of dementia.

People with Dementia

For many people with dementia and their caregivers, the home represents their life accomplishments; it is almost always the environment of choice for as long as possible. Although the majority of people with dementia do live at home, this becomes increasingly difficult as the disease progresses, and alternative solutions often become necessary.

Although the progression of Alzheimer's disease is gradual, the solutions for accommodation are not. Since most localities have only "home" or "institutional" options, many people with dementia find themselves in long-term care facilities prematurely. Alternatives, such as day care centers (Sands & Suzuki 1983) or group homes, are not available in many communities and still do not meet all the needs of people with dementia or their caregivers. This

Needs and Goals

People with Dementia

- *Strong emotional ties to "home"*

- *Gradual and variable progression of the disease*

- *Inability to undertake new learning and difficulty adjusting to relocation* necessitates the development of a greater range of environments along the continuum between home and institutional long-term care.

To some extent, the specific losses incurred at each stage of AD vary among individuals; people with dementia may also lose competencies in some areas while retaining them in others. More restrictive and institutional environments tend to assume total dependency on the part of people with dementia and do not, for the most part, allow the exercise of remaining competencies. This often results in the phenomenon of "excess disability" in the person with dementia (Kahn 1975). Although support is needed in areas of decreasing or lost competence, stimulation and challenge can and should continue in realms where higher competence remains. The necessary amount of increased control and support is determined by the individual decrease in autonomy.

Because people with dementia are quite limited in the amount of new information that they can incorporate, relocation from setting to setting can be confusing and should be limited when possible. Campus arrangements that contain a variety of settings in close proximity, sharing many services, spaces, and staff members, are one way to resolve much of this relocation trauma. For example, a person with dementia could live in a variety of facilities throughout the progression of the disease (e.g., assisted-living apartment to group home to long-term care facility) while continuing to use the same outdoor park and wandering path, visit the same clinic and major activity areas, and work with the same music director and physical therapist.

Needs of Caregivers

Needs of Caregivers

• *A spectrum of services and environmental options*

Life as a caregiver can be debilitating, and family members are often described as the second victims of Alzheimer's disease. Because of the very limited range of available environmental options (fig. 2.1), family caregivers are often forced to choose between the overwhelming burden of caring for the person with dementia alone at home and the guilt and frustration of accepting institutionalization before this may be necessary. A greater range of settings and increased availability of services for caregivers and people with dementia can extend the time during which each environmental option is feasible (e.g., a longer stay with a spouse in an apartment in a shared housing arrangement before moving to a long-term care facility).

Figure 2.1
Potential environmental accommodations can be related to the stages of dementia during which they are most often used.

Stages of Alzheimer's Disease	Living with family			Living away from home		
	House	Shared Housing	Day Care	Group Home	Long-term care	Hospice
Stage I	////	////	////	////		
Stage 2		////	////	////	////	
Stage 3					////	////

Organizational Needs

Facilities for people with dementia must be responsive to the changing characteristics of this population, in terms of both varying representation of the three stages of the disease and decreasing capabilities of the resident population over time. To limit resident turnover and to secure a broader economic base, which are in the best interests of the facility, environments for people with dementia should be able to provide for more than a single, narrowly-defined stage of the disease at a given time.

Therapeutic Goals

Options along a continuum of care can help to blur the sharp boundaries that currently exist between different facility types and can introduce additional variations. For example, more homelike units in long-term care facilities are a possible new alternative to the familiar large nursing unit. Such developments will help to retain ties with the healthy and the familiar that are often lost in the move to a traditional institutional setting.

It is important to support the highest level of functional ability of people with dementia. Both Mace (1987) and Peppard (1986) emphasized the importance of supporting those abilities not totally impaired by dementia to enhance the sense of competence and self-esteem. People with dementia should be provided with regulated stimulation and challenge in response to their remaining capabilities. The availability of several options along a continuum of care permits adaptation to the changing needs and capabilities of people with dementia. More generally, a responsive continuum of care requires that all settings along the continuum respond to more of the needs of people with dementia and their caregivers.

Common Existing Options

The home is presently the most common setting for people with dementia. The majority of older persons, like other Americans, live in detached single-family houses that they own. Possible interventions in this setting occur at the micro-scale and typically include things like labeling drawers to aid in orientation, installing grab bars for negotiability, or installing a gate to enclose a backyard for security. At times, a second floor might become inaccessible, necessitating the conversion of a first floor room or the creation of an additional space to provide for better supervision of people with dementia. In this instance, the unused upstairs room can be converted to a private "retreat" for the caregiver; having such a space may help to alleviate some the stress associated with this role. Services such as housekeeping and in-home day care can also help to make the home a viable alternative for the caregiver and the person with dementia for an extended period.

In response to increasing demands on caregivers at home, day care facilities provide alternative environments for people with dementia for periods extending from a few hours to a full day. Day care facilities might become even more useful by beginning to offer occasional overnight respite services, thereby al-

Organizational Needs

- *Provision for a changing population and changing characteristics of people with dementia*

Therapeutic Goals

- *Retain ties to the healthy and familiar.*
- *Adapt to the changing needs and capabilities of people with dementia.*
- *Consider all other therapeutic goals.*

Policy, Planning, and Design Concepts

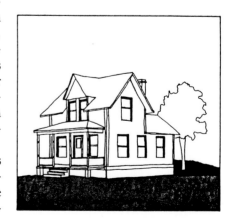

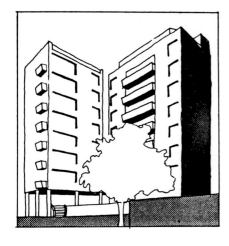

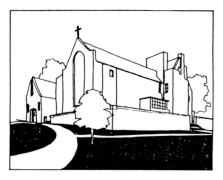

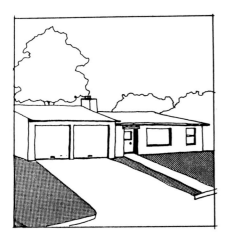

lowing the spouse or members of the family to go away for the weekend while leaving the person with dementia in a familiar and comforting environment. Some day care facilities are beginning to offer personal grooming services. The task of assisting the person with dementia to bathe or shower is often overwhelming, especially when the family caregiver is a frail, elderly spouse. Bathing can often be accomplished more safely and easily by professional day care staff members. Extension of the hours that day care is available to correspond with traditional working hours (e.g., 8:00 a.m. to 6:00 p.m. instead of 10:00 a.m. to 4:00 p.m.) might also make it possible for the family caregiver to continue to work while the person with dementia lives at home.

Group homes are another existing option along the continuum of care, although they are relatively limited in number at present. These are most often existing houses within the community, modified to accommodate a small group of residents and one or two caregivers. Group homes might be situated in a "cottage" type arrangement, so that a number of group homes could share amenities like a common outdoor area and wandering path, exercise facilities, a small clinic, and other services and spaces. Group homes could also affiliate with a particular long-term care facility to take advantage of its specialized staff and services.

Care must be taken to maintain the domestic and familiar atmosphere that is characteristic of group homes, situated as they usually are in renovated single-family dwellings. There is a danger that staff members and designers more familiar with institutional settings will create "mini-nursing homes" in the group home. The addition of a nurses' station in the front hall of one group home is such a device.

Most often housed in nursing homes or hospitals for the chronically ill, long-term care facilities are characterized by the traditions of the "medical model," with a focus on care-giving and supervision. There is a great potential for such settings to become more homelike and familiar through such means as the use of residential furnishings and fixtures, the promotion of autonomy and independence for people with dementia in the accomplishment of activities of daily living, and the adoption of policies and activities that will preserve the dignity and promote the self-esteem of residents. Many nursing homes could extend the continuum of care by offering services such as day care and respite care to people with dementia in the community.

Creating New Options

Environments for people with dementia are defined by both the physical setting and the range of services that they offer. Different combinations of several building forms (single-family homes, congregate housing, group homes, nursing homes) together with the provision of various services (prepared meals, housekeeping, day care, assistance with personal care) can provide new options for people at different stages of Alzheimer's disease (see fig. 2.2).

Other entirely new types of environments could be developed. These might be designed to complement existing options. Assisted living apartments for people with dementia and their spouses are an attractive alternative; these might be located adjacent to the long-term care facility and might offer such

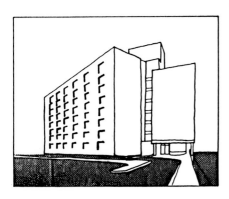

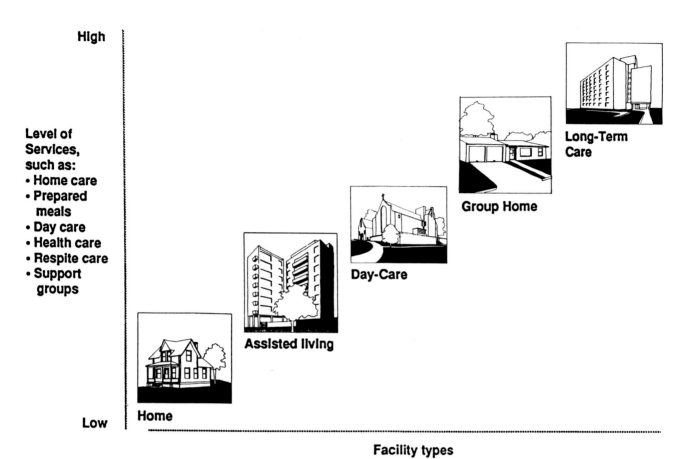

Figure 2.2
This schematic diagram illustrates the relationships between level of services and environmental options. For example, more services can be offered to people with dementia living at home to extend their stay in the community; environmental modifications and a less institutional image can bring a long-term care facility closer to home. (After Lawton 1987.)

services as housekeeping, access to day care and community dining facilities, and special activities and spaces (e.g., a club house and a miniature golf course) for the spouses of people with dementia. These would make it possible for the person with dementia and the caregiver to remain together in a more supportive environment that included some building services (e.g., a "call button" to reach a professional staff member in emergencies, weekly housekeeping service, a day care center in the basement).

Campus arrangements, similar to existing senior housing villages, are another relatively unexplored option. These could offer the entire continuum of services and settings for people with dementia and their caregivers. Minimal assistance apartments could be included; these could continue to be occupied by the caregiver even after a move by the person with dementia. Day care, a group home for persons with more advanced Alzheimer's disease, a site for activities and support group meetings for spouses, and a long-term care setting, perhaps adjacent to a clinic, small grocery store, hairdresser, and other convenient amenities, should also be included in this type of arrangement.

Figure 2.3
This facility does not possess the traditional monolithic structure of a medium-sized nursing home; instead, it is organized in a series of smaller units that look like homes and are operated like autonomous households. (Drawing after Woodside Place, Oakmont, Pa.; Perkins, Geddes, Eastman, Architects.)

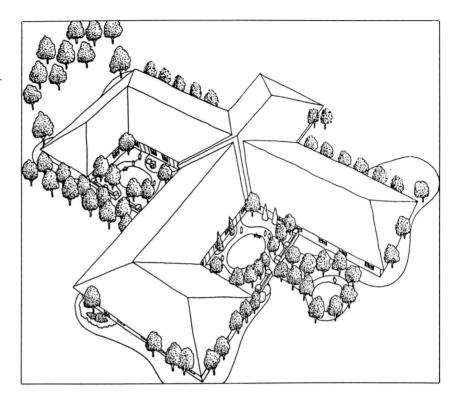

Holding On to Home

There are two ways in which the fundamental theme of "holding on to home" may be applied to policy, planning, and design. First, various combinations of services and environmental modifications can make it possible for people with dementia to remain comfortably at home for much longer than is common now. In this sense, adaptations make it possible for people with dementia literally to "hold on to home." Second, the qualities of "home" and the normalized life patterns that they imply should be extended to other types of environments wherever possible. In this way, nondomestic settings could acquire some of the characteristics of the home environment which have a positive influence on people with dementia (fig. 2.3).

A responsive continuum of care including a range of options can provide the least restrictive environments for people with dementia. By striking a balance between organizational and community support on one hand and the highest level of independence for persons with dementia and their caregivers on the other, autonomy, control, and the dignity of both can be maintained.

Related Principles   Tapping Local Resources 2.2

Planning environments for people with dementia requires consideration of both the services and the physical setting to be provided. Not all services need be provided on site because the surrounding community probably provides a system of such services, which constitute a valuable resource in both economic and therapeutic terms. Tapping local resources can eliminate unnecessary and expensive duplication of services and maintain beneficial links with the community.

2.2 Tapping Local Resources

People with Dementia

The needs of people with dementia and their caregivers obviously vary with facility type and the capabilities of the population being served. In addition to the generalized provision of care, there may be a need for information and professional consultation, support for continued residence at home, therapeutic activities for residents, social activities for caregivers, or medical services. For example, a group home for people in the early stages of dementia may benefit from access to activities at a local senior center, health clinic, or music school.

Organizational Needs

Facility administrators must assess the availability of additional community resources, such as an adequate pool of potential employees and transportation access for staff, family, and friends.

Therapeutic Goals

Facilities for people with dementia must respond to both major variations in needs across individuals and variations within individuals over time. Access to a broad system of services and resources can provide this necessary adaptability.

Like everyone else, people with dementia are likely to have accumulated a lifetime of experiences and associations from their active years of living within the community. Facilities that are able to tap local resources and maintain links with the community assist people with dementia in retaining ties to the healthy and familiar.

Inventory and Integration of Resources in the Facility Program

In planning a facility at any point along the continuum of care, it is essential to develop an inventory of services and resources available in the community. Services potentially valuable to people with dementia and their caregivers include information and consultation (referral for services, counseling, and legal and financial assistance); support for people living at home (visiting and phone reassurance, home-delivered meals, housekeeping assistance, at-home medical care, transportation); and therapy and medical care. In addition, parks, theaters, museums, and shopping centers—though not traditional

---

Needs and Goals

People with Dementia

- *There is typically a need for a broad range of medical, social, and other professional services.*

Therapeutic Goals

- *Respond to changing needs of people with dementia.*
- *Maintain ties with the healthy and familiar.*

Policy, Planning, and Design Concepts

community "services"—can be valuable resources for people in the middle stages of dementia.

Potential Community Services

Information and Referral

Families of people with dementia need information about the disease and about the options and sources of support available to them within the community. Information and referral services may be provided by local chapters of the Alzheimer's Association, a local senior center, or family support groups.

Home-delivered Meals

Patients unable to shop or prepare their own meals might benefit from a service providing home-delivered meals.

Respite Care

Caregivers of people with dementia need occasional relief or respite from the stress of caregiving. Respite care, from a few hours a week to several months a year, might be provided by volunteers from a local church or senior citizen center or by trained home care agency staff.

Home Care

Many families find that they are able to maintain a person with dementia at home longer if they have in-home assistance in the provision of care. Services range from supervision and help with household maintenance to the provision of such specialized health services as nursing care, speech therapy, and occupational therapy.

Family Support Groups

Family support groups are composed of the friends and relatives of Alzheimer's patients who meet regularly to share information and discuss common problems. They offer caregivers a chance to share encouragement, support, and understanding with others coping with similar difficulties.

Individual and Family Counseling

Counseling by private practitioners or in clinic settings may be necessary for families that require support beyond that provided by support groups, families, or friends.

Legal and Financial Advice

Alzheimer's disease often leads to the need for long-term care. This raises a range of legal and financial issues for spouses and families, which might necessitate services provided by law firms or legal agencies specializing in Alzheimer's disease.

Location

Locational decisions are likely to have far-reaching implications for the design and functioning of a facility for people with dementia. While there are no data demonstrating the superiority of one location over another, it might reasonably be hypothesized that populated urban settings may create conditions of high sensory stimulation or even overload, whereas more remote rural locations may limit maintenance of existing community ties (fig. 2.4).

Currently, decisions regarding the locations of environments for people with dementia seem to be a consequence of land availability and/or proximity to related facilities. Thus, it is essential to identify those therapeutic and organizational goals that seem to be most appropriate for a particular facility type and then to identify a location that maximizes the utilization of those resources judged most important. Suburban locations may provide additional outdoor space and proximity to family caregivers but may be more remote from medical and cultural facilities or the largest pool of potential employees. It is important to ensure easy access, rather than just proximity, particularly for staff, some of whom may need to rely on public transportation networks.

Capitalizing on Site Opportunities

Each type of specialized facility for people with dementia has its own requirements with respect to location and site development. For day care facilities, easy vehicular and pedestrian accessibility is important, as is proximity to clients' homes. Group homes should be characterized by domestic imagery and located within residential neighborhoods. Accessibility to outdoor spaces is also a desirable feature (fig. 2.5); even though residents are not allowed out unchaperoned, proximity to retail and other community facilities can open up new possibilities for meaningful activities. For long-term care facilities, outdoor areas and their incorporation into the facility are very important, taking precedence over considerations such as access.

Maximizing Opportunities for Family Contact

Recognizing the importance of family visits in the lives of people with dementia, it is important to identify those factors that can increase visiting by family members, such as easy access to the facility. It is equally important to recognize and respond to less obvious influences. For example, the provision of appropriate activities can make visiting meaningful for people with dementia and their families and friends. The overall image of the facility should also be welcoming and noninstitutional. Organizational policies might include introduction of a shuttle service to make visiting more convenient.

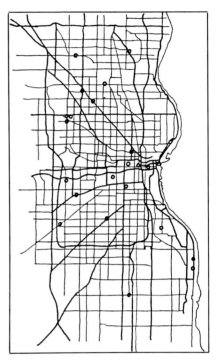

Figure 2.4
Day care and related facilities distributed across a metropolitan region may be viewed as a system of services.

Responsive Continuum of Care 2.1

Related Principles

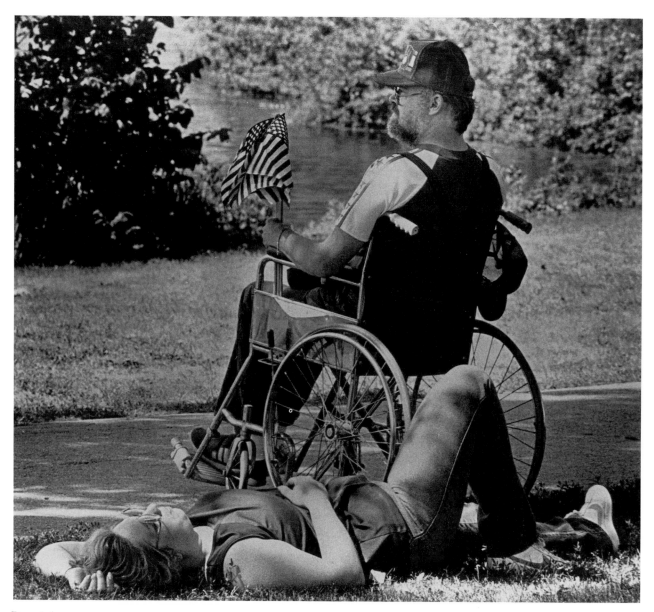

Figure 2.5
Local parks can provide unique opportunities for recreation, contact with the natural environment, and celebration of holidays. (Jerry and Pat Schmidt, photographed by Susie Post.)

2.3 Appropriate Group Size

Determination of facility size and of the numbers of caregivers and people to be served is one of the earliest and most important decisions in the development of facilities for people with dementia. In the past, such decisions were typically based upon pragmatic considerations such as available space, staffing, and budget. However, there is increasing evidence to suggest that group size may have significant behavioral and psychological consequences for people with dementia. To the extent possible, both organizational and architectural environments should be designed to ensure that people with dementia feel that they are a part of a small (rather than a large) group.

People with Dementia

The influence of group size on people with dementia can be readily understood. Relocation from one's home to any group setting involves major discontinuities in social, organizational, and physical aspects of the environment. It involves getting used to living in a group situation and dealing with large numbers of people, a situation that can be difficult for the most competent population. Residents may be easily overwhelmed by a complex and unfamiliar setting (Peppard 1986). The situation is further complicated by the fact that people with dementia experience a declining ability to adapt to varying environmental demands (Hall & Buckwalter 1986).

Smaller group sizes can make group living more manageable for people with dementia as anonymity is reduced. Such a noninstitutional and family-like environment could encourage more visitation by family and friends by allowing the establishment of social ties between unrelated families of residents who might belong to the same small group or "household."

Organizational Needs

Newly emerging facilities (such as boarding homes) are by definition small in scale, with a maximum of eight to a dozen residents. Other facilities (such as special care units within long-term care facilities) may vary dramatically in size, with the smallest accommodating ten or twelve residents and the largest up to fifty (Ohta & Ohta 1988). Although there is only limited research data, professionals seem to agree that unit size may have significant therapeutic impact. Ohta and Ohta (1988, 804) suggest that smaller special care units appear to "promote friendships and socialization among patients, and foster a sense of neighborhood." Such characteristics, they suggest, are not present in the largest of units, where "patients are presented with a large and highly variable set of social stimuli, making the feeling of intimacy extremely difficult to achieve."

Similarly, variations in staffing ratios also influence the sense of belonging to a group for people with dementia. Among a sample of special care units, staff to patient ratios range from a low of 1:12 during the day shift and 1:25 on the night shift to a high of 1:3. Higher ratios contribute to a greater sense of belonging, as people with dementia then relate to fewer staff at a more personal level. Here again, organizational decisions about staffing ratios seem to have therapeutic consequences.

Therapeutic Goals

To the extent that people with dementia feel a part of a small group, it is likely that their ties with familiar home environments will be strengthened. This

Needs and Goals

People with Dementia

- *Complex and unfamiliar environments may become increasingly overwhelming.*

Therapeutic Goals

- *Maximize ties to the healthy and familiar.*

- *Increase opportunities for socialization.*
- *Regulate degrees of sensory and social stimulation.*

can facilitate the maintenance of normal social roles for people with dementia (Alvermann 1979; Coons 1985).

Smaller groups can also encourage greater socialization, as people with dementia are not overwhelmed by the unfamiliarity of large numbers of people. Additionally, small groups are likely to provide regulated stimulation and to be less stressful for people with dementia, who may be unable to handle the stimulation and stress associated with transition to a group living situation.

Policy, Planning, and Design Concepts

Group size is typically defined in terms of the number of people with dementia under the supervision of a number of staff and caregivers (e.g., the number of residents in a nursing unit in a long-term care facility). While desirable, it is not always possible to create facilities with small numbers of users and high staffing ratios. To meet therapeutic goals, however, it is desirable and possible to break these functional groups into smaller groups through both organizational and architectural means (fig. 2.6).

Consistent Contact

Staff in special care units (typically those with high staff to patient ratios) consistently deal with the same patients and "are adamant in their belief that such (consistent) staffing is essential" (Ohta & Ohta 1988, 805). Little or no reported staff stress and turnover in special care units with high staff to patient ratios serves to enhance further the consistency of staffing.

Consistency of contact for people with dementia is enhanced through continuing interaction with the same individuals. The friendships, socialization, and sense of neighborhood observed in smaller special care units reflect the ability of each resident "to see and interact with a small and constant set of other patients throughout the day, each and every day" (Ohta & Ohta 1988, 804).

Small Residential Clusters

Architecturally, small social groupings may be defined through the clustering of resident rooms and some associated activity areas (fig. 2.7). Within long-term care facilities, such clusters should consist of eight to sixteen residents.

Figure 2.6
The concept of residential clusters is extended into a day care facility. Living, dining, and kitchen areas accommodate smaller groups of people and also reinforce the domestic character of the center. Although each area has a clear architectural identity, there is easy visual and functional access among them.

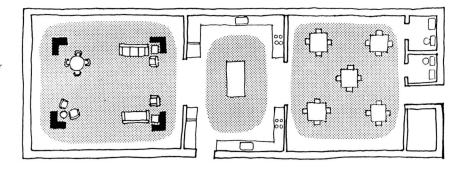

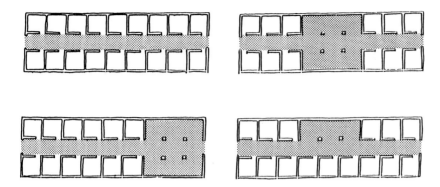

Figure 2.7
Three strategies are illustrated for the creation
of residential clusters within a traditional
twenty-four-resident long-term care unit. The
open spaces created eliminate the long corridor
with identical doors on either side and accom-
modate dining and other functions that are
brought into the unit.

With respect to daily activities, these clusters may be self-contained, accommodating all functions, including dining. Employing design and planning strategies that introduce "living rooms," "dining rooms," and their associated activities further reinforces the desired "residential" character.

Clusters of Small Activity Spaces 4.1

Related Principles

Overleaf: Hanson Graphic; Ed Held, photographed by Tom Bamberger

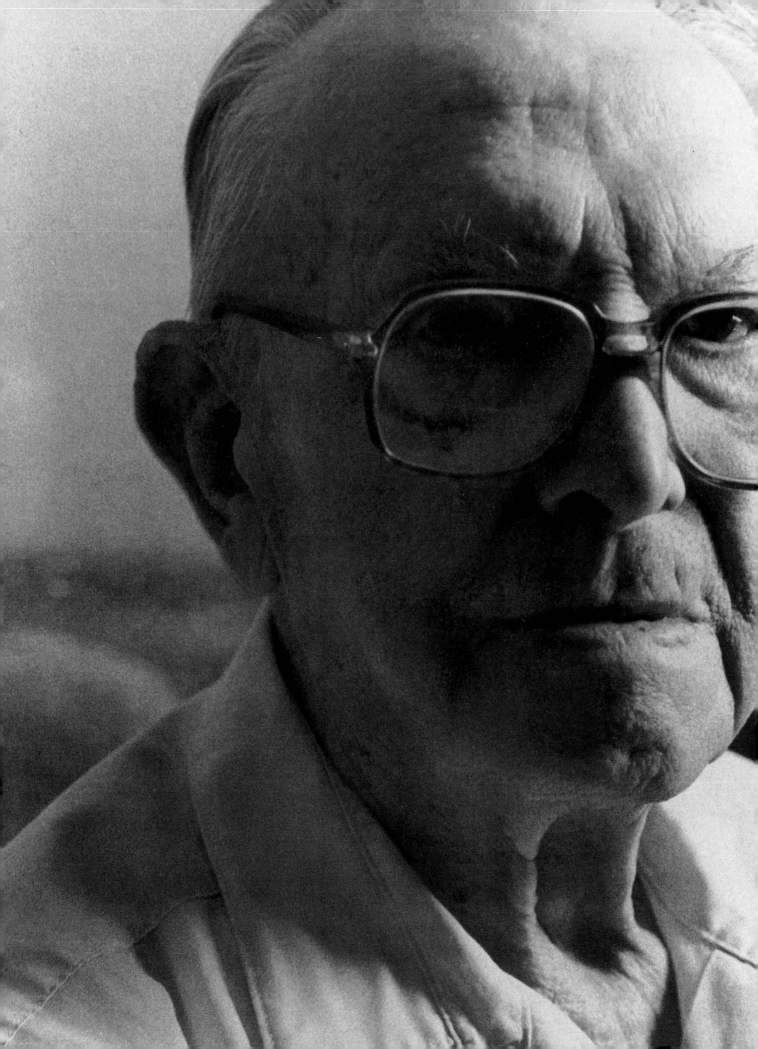

3 *Principles for Design: General Attributes of the Environment*

One's experience of and behavior in a particular environment are influenced not only by specific architectural features or elements but also by more general qualities or attributes of that setting. In the planning and design of environments for people with dementia, four such attributes seem to be particularly salient: image, negotiability, familiarity, and stimulation. In each case, it is important to remember that, while these attributes are a function of the physical environment, they also reflect the interactions of physical, organizational, and social subsystems. Thus, creation of a more "homelike" environment is the consequence of appropriate furnishings and finishes, patterns of ongoing behavior typical of those found in residential settings, and policies and programs supportive of such residential activities.

Principles for design in this section address pervasive characteristics of the environment that will influence and often dictate the design of specific individual spaces within the facility or home environment. For example, the principle Eliminating Environmental Barriers *recommends such design strategies as multiple cueing to reinforce environmental messages (e.g., signs, furnishings, and good food smells to indicate the function of the dining room), which can be used throughout the facility to designate and characterize particular spaces. The principle* Things from the Past *advocates reminiscence to strengthen ties to the healthy and familiar and maintain long-term memory among residents; this recommendation can be translated into design decisions that will affect the furnishings and character of a facility for people with dementia, as well as the activities in which residents engage (e.g., familiar and meaningful activities such as baking cookies or folding laundry) and organizational policies (e.g., the practice of residents bringing some personal possessions from home to furnish bedrooms and public areas).*

3.1 Noninstitutional Character

Even in the largest facilities for people with dementia, there are planning and design strategies that can minimize "institutional" character, maximize domestic qualities, and lead people to feel that this is a place where they "belong." Domestic ambience goes beyond elements such as drapes or upholstered chairs. Organizational issues that provide residents with a measure of autonomy and control over their lives can significantly contribute to a noninstitutional environment.

Needs and Goals

People with Dementia

- *People with dementia, like other people, are most familiar with conventional residential settings.*

People with Dementia

Treatment facilities and residential environments for people with dementia often possess "institutional" characteristics that are viewed negatively by family, friends, and staff, as well as by people with dementia themselves. Physical design often responds only to practical and economical delivery of care, manifested in long institutional corridors, spaces with standardized fixtures and equipment, and a nonresidential character. Group sizes tend to be considerably larger than those with which most people are familiar and comfortable, further reinforcing an institutional character. Stimulation is frequently absent or there is a surfeit of it, either of which can be counter-therapeutic for people with dementia. Some of the confusion, disorientation, and discomfort experienced as a consequence of these negative institutional characteristics may be minimized by creating environments that are more familiar, homelike, and noninstitutional in character.

Therapeutic Goals

- *Maintain ties with the healthy and familiar.*

- *Regulate levels of sensory stimulation.*

- *Maximize autonomy and control.*

Therapeutic Goals

To the extent possible, environments for people with dementia should assist them in maintaining ties to that with which they are familiar and comfortable. Even a facility that is part of a large institution can be patterned after the outside community and develop its own domestic identity and character.

Institutional environments are often characterized by a virtual absence of either sensory or social stimulation, with people sitting passively in large undifferentiated spaces often with rows and rows of side-by-side seating lined up against a long wall. Conversely, the presence of large numbers of other people can result in overstimulation. The goal should therefore be regulation and variation of stimulation to ensure that it is both manageable and interesting for people with dementia (Lawton 1981; Mace 1987).

There is a danger that large institutions will treat clients or residents in a nonindividualized fashion. To the extent possible, people with dementia should retain opportunities for personal control and individual expression.

Design Concepts

Human Scale

Institutional environments often comprise large, unbroken building masses that overwhelm the people who live in or use them. Externally, this institutional character can be broken down by creating a larger number of smaller building pieces (figs. 3.1 and 3.2). Internally, this can likewise be achieved by breaking down the organizational (as well as the physical) structure of the environment through the creation of small groups as well as small, clearly identifiable spaces.

Avoidance of "Hard Architecture"

Institutional environments were characterized by Sommer (1974) as "hard architecture"—built from materials such as ceramic tile, plastic laminate, and stainless steel, which were meant to be indestructible. Recognizing the

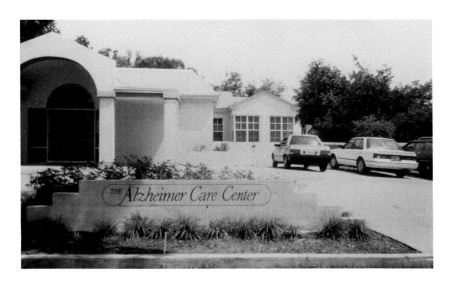

Figure 3.1
The entry to this day care center retains many of the characteristics of a residential building. The entry serves to reduce the apparent size of the facility. (Alzheimer Care Center, Orlando, Fla.)

needs of hygiene and maintenance, it is still possible to minimize the "hard" qualities of environments for people with dementia. This can be done by using current technology and new materials (e.g., moisture-resistant fabric in lieu of vinyl upholstery) that are efficient and durable and yet retain some domestic qualities (fig. 3.3).

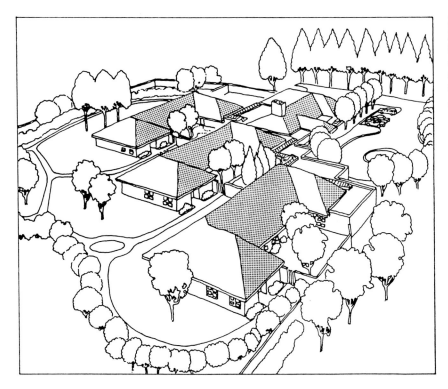

Figure 3.2
Location surrounded by trees, separation of the building into "house-like" forms, shingle roof, and wooden siding all serve to enhance the human scale and noninstitutional character of this facility. (Drawing after Woodside Place, Oakmont, Pa.; Perkins, Geddes, Eastman, Architects.)

Figure 3.3
The presence of books, the brick hearth, and
skylights all help to keep "hard architecture" to
a minimum.

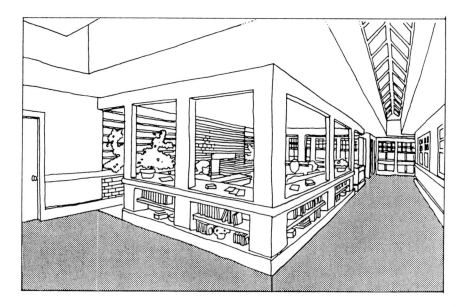

Variation within Common Themes

Institutions are a paradox in that they often present either a surfeit or a lack of stimulation. On the one hand, large undifferentiated spaces with too many people and loud intercoms are not uncommon; at the same time, repetitiveness, standardization, and uniformity in fixtures, furnishings, and architectural character are also common in many such settings. It is important to "regulate" these extremes and to make the level of stimulation both comprehensible and manageable for people with dementia (fig. 3.4).

Related Principles

Things from the Past 3.3
Entry and Transition 5.1
Domestic Kitchens 5.3

3.2 Eliminating Environmental Barriers

Physical and cognitive impairments associated with dementia often make using and moving through the environment difficult. It is imperative to eliminate barriers to negotiability in environments for people with dementia. In addition to traditional solutions such as ramps or handrails, environmental interventions may include clear or consistent information and easy to operate handles and controls.

Needs and Goals

People with Dementia

People with Dementia

Dementing diseases often exacerbate common age-related problems in performing seemingly simple tasks, such as fastening buttons or closing snaps.

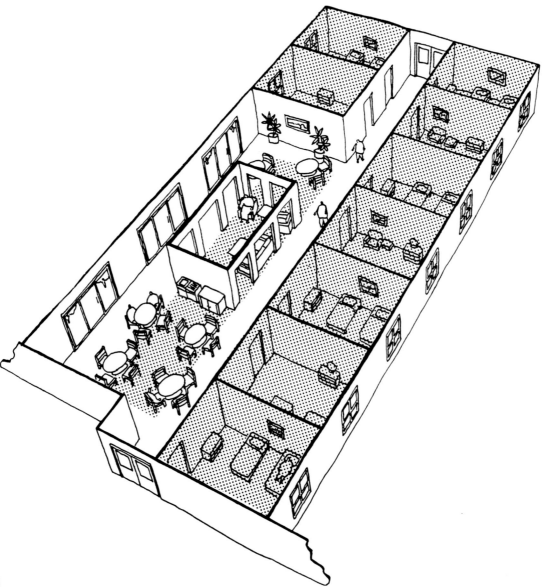

Figure 3.4
The renovation of a typical wing of a long-term care facility replaces one side of a corridor, lined with identical resident rooms, with clearly defined dining and social spaces.

These difficulties reflect a variety of factors, including apraxia, in which messages from the brain are simply not transmitted to the hands and fingers, despite the fact that the person with dementia knows what he or she wants to do; tremors, muscle weakness, and joint and bone diseases, such as arthritis; and vision problems, such as difficulty differentiating similar color intensities (Mace & Rabins 1981). The individual's awareness of the difficulties being experienced creates a vicious cycle in which resulting tension, worry, and embarrassment are further obstacles to performance.

• *Concerns about performance may make people with dementia hesitant to take on tasks.*

Therapeutic Goals

- *Ensure safety and security.*

- *Support highest level of functional ability.*

- *Maximize opportunities for autonomy and control.*

Design Concepts

Therapeutic Goals

As a consequence of the range of impairments that people with dementia are likely to experience, the environment may present barriers to effective use and movement. To ensure safety and security of clients and residents, these barriers should be eliminated to facilitate easy negotiation of the environment.

The level of functional ability of people with dementia is likely to be enhanced through the mitigation of environmental barriers and hazards. Enhanced accessibility and negotiability can help maintain residents' sense of autonomy and control.

Because of turnover in client population and of progression through the disease, environments for people with dementia typically must contend with changing resident needs. At any one time, various stages of the disease are likely to be represented; therefore, it is essential to respond to these several stages and to ensure negotiability for all segments of the population.

Multiple Sensory Cueing

Presenting the same information in multiple ways through redundant cueing reinforces environmental messages and increases the likelihood of their being perceived and understood (Pastalan 1979). Redundant cueing might include the use of olfactory as well as visual cues; the aroma of cooking foods can provide a powerful olfactory cue for finding the kitchen or dining room (fig. 3.5). Even when only one sensory modality is used for cueing, it is possible to employ more than one device. Redundant cueing could make the entrance to a resident's room more identifiable through the use of a distinctive color and photographs, as well as by providing a memorable name plate.

Figure 3.5
Placing the kitchen in an open and visible area, rather than behind walls, facilitates recognition through multiple sensory cues. Residents are then more likely to find the kitchen because they can see it and also smell cooking from the corridor, as well as hear the clatter of dishes and mealtime conversation.

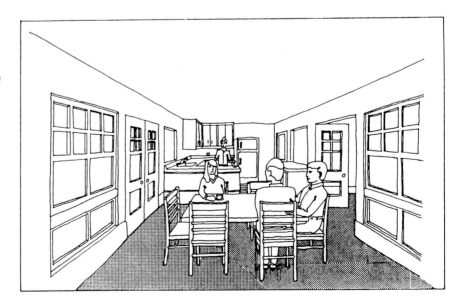

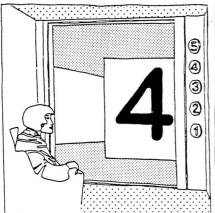

Figure 3.6
Location of signage at a consistant height and location helps people know where to look for needed information. In this example, the floor number is always located at the same spot, where it is visible from the elevator. Residents can learn where to look for this information.

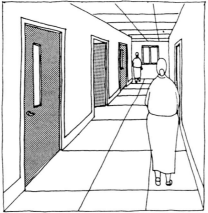

Figure 3.7
Only doorways to resident rooms are accentuated for identification. Doors to service spaces are made to appear as inconspicuous as possible.

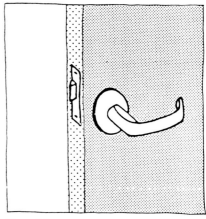

Figure 3.8
Lever action door handles, large controls on telephones, and extended arms on easy chairs all compensate for decreased capabilities.

Consistent Messages

The environment should communicate information in a consistent way (fig. 3.6). For example, the color red may be associated with "hot" and blue with "cold." Such consistent repetition of color coding can introduce an important element of predictability and order into an environment.

Accentuation of the Message, with Moderate Background Stimulation

By reducing the stimulus value of the background to a minimum—for example, by using a contrasting color only for those doors used by clients or residents—information for orientation can be communicated with greater clarity (fig. 3.7).

Compensatory Design

Often, objects in the environment can be designed to compensate for the decreased capabilities (e.g., hand-eye coordination or visual acuity) of people with dementia. Lever action handles are far easier to operate than door knobs (fig. 3.8), as are pressure plate light controls instead of the common switch and telephones with larger and more legible push buttons. It should be borne in mind, however, that new learning is unlikely for people with dementia; thus, these designs should not require new learning or their compensatory function may not be fulfilled.

Koncelik (1976) suggested "self-correcting" design as an approach that can facilitate as well as guide and correct movements of people with dementia. One example is locks with recessed tumblers to guide the key into the tumbler.

| Related Principles | Dignified Bathing 5.7 |

3.3 Things from the Past

Familiar artifacts, activities, and environments can provide valuable associations with the past for people with dementia and can stimulate opportunities for social interaction and meaningful activity. Rather than being limited to a single "rummage box," the total environment can potentially serve to trigger reminiscence.

Needs and Goals

People with Dementia

- *Emotional components of memory may be retained even after the loss of other components.*

Therapeutic Goals

- *Retain ties with the healthy and familiar.*

- *Support the highest level of functional ability.*

- *Create opportunities for socialization.*

People with Dementia

While people with dementia cannot remember or be taught to remember recent events (Gwyther 1986), their long-term memory—especially the emotional components—remains relatively intact until the later stages of the disease. Things from the past can stimulate the exercise and celebration of these remaining capabilities.

Therapeutic Goals

Artifacts and things from the past can add to the creation of familiar environments to which people with dementia can more readily adapt (fig. 3.9). Such objects can serve as a means of maintaining orientation to time and place that is less formalized than traditional "reality orientation" (Folsom 1983), which is typically restricted to a board listing facility name, date, and weather information (Barnes 1974).

Familiar activities and the reinstatement of meaningful social roles (Coons 1985) can support remaining functional abilities and enhance a sense of competence. Opportunities for reminiscence that encourage residents to reflect on their pasts can serve to initiate contact between residents and promote increased socialization.

Design Concepts

Spaces for Familiar Tasks

Spaces should be provided for supporting activities that are familiar to residents. Such activities might include cooking, baking cookies (fig. 3.10), and gardening. A central outdoor island with room for several residents to engage in a variety of activities around raised planters (permitting access from a seated position or from a wheelchair) is one way to support such activities. Places for familiar activities should be both visible and accessible to residents to provide orientational cues and also to encourage participation, both active and passive.

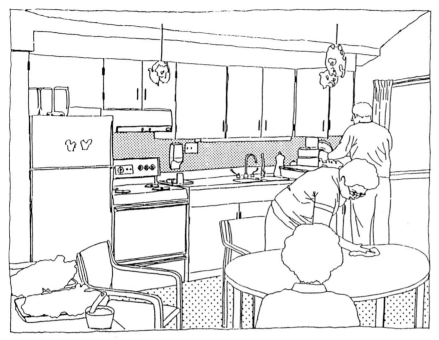

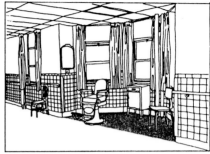

Figure 3.9
Male residents receive their daily shave in this barber's chair located in an alcove adjacent to a major corridor. It is a highly visible activity with powerful personal associations.

Figure 3.10
Familiar and common activities are also a trigger for reminiscence. A simple activity such as baking cookies can evoke associations with the past and foster social interactions.

Museum

Actual artifacts and objects from residents' pasts can be gathered together to form a museum. Such a museum might be anything from a display case along a corridor (fig. 3.11) to a series of rooms displaying objects from the past (fig. 3.12); it could be centralized or dispersed. Functionally, it might range from stage sets that one could passively observe to activity areas for actual use.

Familiar Places, Familiar People

By being visible and accessible, familiar things from residents' pasts can serve as landmarks, facilitating orientation among people with dementia. Family albums containing photographs of family members and important life events could trigger reminiscence and initiate conversation in otherwise inactive residents. They could also facilitate orientation with regard to person, helping people with dementia know who they are and serving as a reassurance device for residents between visitations. A family album can help caregivers learn about the unique histories and pasts of people with dementia and enhance staff understanding and recognition of residents. Photographic displays and video cassettes can be used for the same purpose (fig. 3.13).

Policy Implications

The creation of a more familiar, legible, and personalized environment can be facilitated if people with dementia are allowed to bring some of their own belongings and furniture with them. This has clear implications for environ-

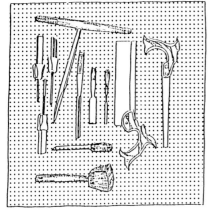

Figure 3.11
This case along a busy corridor displays historic farm tools of great personal significance to residents of the surrounding farming community.

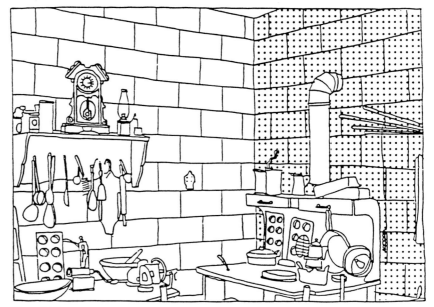

Figure 3.12
This arrangement of a turn-of-the-century kitchen is a favored area within a "museum" created in a long-term facility.

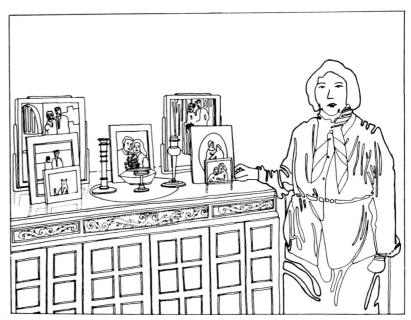

Figure 3.13
A variety of images—from family pictures, both recent and older, to the picture of a favorite cat—can trigger reminiscence. The media are not limited to still photography: movies and video displays can be used as well.

mental design because activity spaces and resident rooms should not therefore be designed only for built-in furniture.

While accommodation and inclusion of artifacts from the past may counter traditional images of a "well-ordered" environment, it is important to recognize their potential for improving the quality of life of people with dementia. At the same time, staff must be aware that the inclusion of too many artifacts/objects can cause clutter and thereby compromise legibility and safety.

Noninstitutional Character 3.1
Domestic Kitchens 5.3
Places for Visiting 5.9

Related Principles

Sensory and social stimulation in environments for people with dementia (day care facilities, group homes, long-term care facilities) should not differ dramatically from that encountered in domestic environments. People with dementia should not be presented with situations of either sensory deprivation or overstimulation. Both physical and organizational environments can be designed to regulate stimulation, providing interest and challenge without becoming overwhelming. Opportunities should be provided for increasing or reducing the level of stimulation to respond to changing needs and tolerance levels of people with dementia over the course of the day.

3.4 Sensory Stimulation without Stress

People with Dementia

Visual, auditory, and other sensory impairments of general aging may create problems in understanding and coping with the environment (Koncelik 1979). For example, decreased sensitivity to high frequency sounds (presbycusis) makes it more difficult to understand conversation in settings with high levels of background noise. Additionally, Alzheimer's disease and related dementias may further impair the effective processing of information from the environment. Among the memory impairments people with dementia may experience is agnosia, the loss of ability to comprehend the meaning or recognize the importance of various types of sensory stimulation. Seemingly low levels of stimulation (e.g., presence of several people in a room) may be experienced as stressful by people with dementia and may significantly reduce their ability to function (Mace & Rabins 1981). Conversely, it has been suggested (Pynoos & Stacey 1986) that some symptoms of dementia are related to the sensory deprivation of institutional environments, manifested by standardized repetitive environments and lack of variety.

Therapeutic Goals

It is essential that there be effective regulation of the sensory stimulation to which people with dementia are exposed. In Mace's (1987) terms, the goal is

Needs and Goals

People with Dementia

- *Dementia may impair effective processing of information from the environment.*

Therapeutic Goals

- *Provide regulated stimulation and challenge.*

- *Ensure awareness and orientation of people with dementia.*

- *Adapt to changing needs of people with dementia.*

Design Concepts

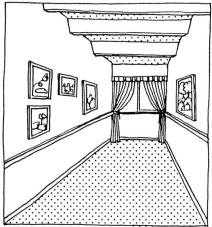

Figure 3.14
The window at the end of the corridor is an unregulated and problematic source of sensory stimulation. The simple addition of a window blind or shade would reduce the problems of glare, too sharp a brightness contrast, and potential disorientation. Similarly, the addition of carpeting would eliminate confusing reflections from the highly polished floor.

one of "stimulation but not stress." Such regulation of stimulation can facilitate the orientation of people with dementia to their physical environment and allow response to changing needs and abilities. Needs and abilities not only change through the course of the disease but may vary over the course of a single day, as tolerance to environmental stimulation varies.

Daily Patterns

Both intensity and content of environmental stimulation may be adjusted over the course of the day in response to changing needs and tolerance levels of people with dementia. The "progressively lowered stress threshold" model of Hall and Buckwalter (1986) modifies levels of environmental stimuli in response to anxiety expressed by people with dementia. As anxious behaviors occur, activities and environmental stimuli are modified and simplified until the anxiety disappears. Large numbers of residents engaging in a wide range of activities can produce considerable stimulation and resultant confusion among people with dementia. Minimizing conflicts between ongoing activities by spatial or temporal separation is an effective way of moderating stimulation. Disruption of temporal patterns (Pynoos & Stacey 1986), referred to commonly as "sundowning," is often associated with dementia. Careful adjustment of stimulation over the course of the day might ensure that people with dementia participate in various activities during the daytime and are sufficiently tired to sleep at night.

Regulation of Stimulation

Environments for people with dementia, like many institutional settings, may be characterized both by very low levels of stimulation (undifferentiated large open spaces and little or no activity) and by overstimulation, as through the use of intercoms and alarms. It is essential to ensure that important environmental messages are effectively communicated to residents. Dampening background noise and enhancing the intensity and target value of various messages may help people with dementia to comprehend their environment. This might be done through the use of carpeting and other sound-absorbing material to moderate background noise and thus enhance speech intelligibility. In addition, dimmer switches, window shades, and doors or partitions are all means for control of the environment and regulation of levels of sensory stimulation (Andreason 1985) (fig. 3.14).

Sensory Involvement Increase

An absence of sensory stimulation can often be just as problematic as too much. Some facilities use textured wall hangings or pieces of carpet, plants, birds, or an aquarium to engage the interest of and encourage exploration by people with dementia (fig. 3.15). Windows are also suggested as a therapeutic tool in institutional environments (Verderber 1982). Additionally, staff behaviors such as touching and handholding can provide increased tactile stimulation and lead to greater involvement between residents and staff.

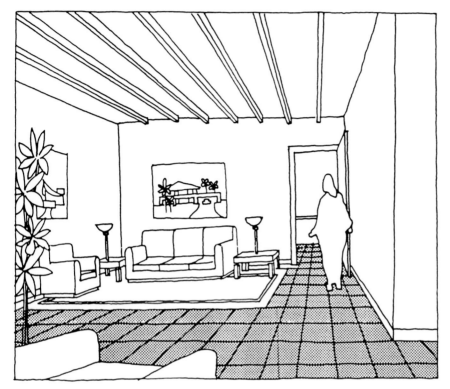

Figure 3.15
Noninstitutional furniture, the homelike use of carpeting and drapes, a beamed ceiling, photographs and paintings on the walls, and the incorporation of natural elements such as plants all contribute to a sense of richness in this day room and enhance the experiential qualities of the setting.

Clusters of Small Activity Spaces 4.1
Public to Private Realms 4.5
Shared Spaces 5.2

Related Principles

Overleaf: Photographed by Tom Bamberger

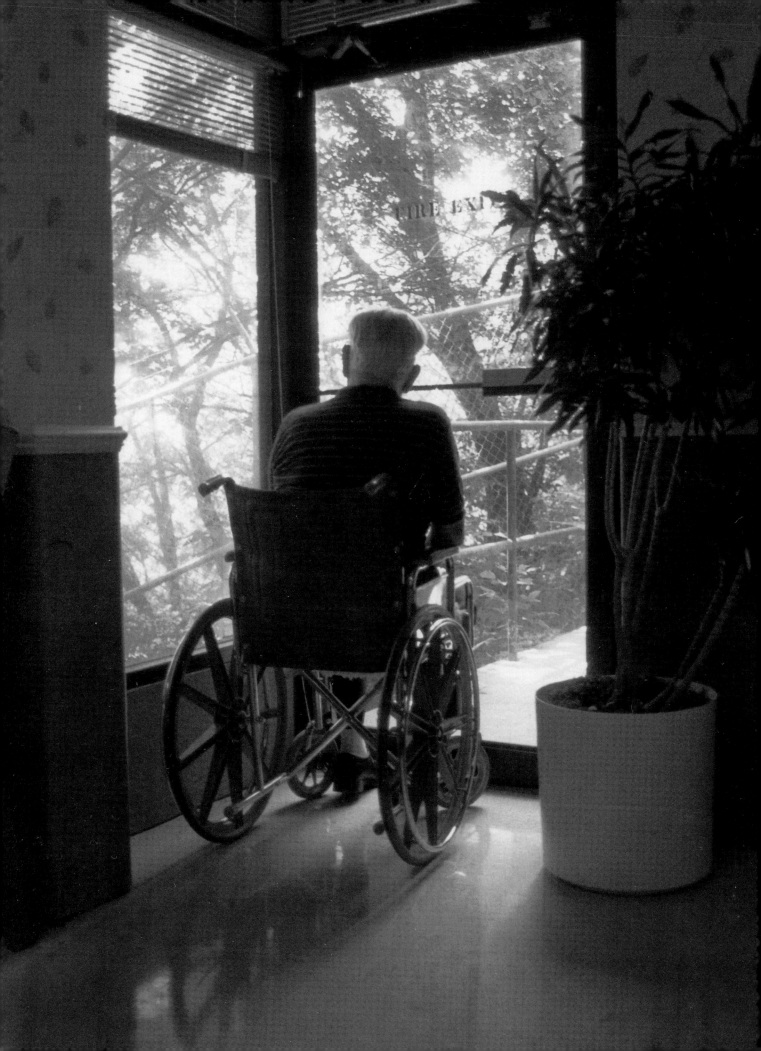

4 Principles for Design: Building Organization

In contrast with preceding principles for design, guidelines in this section are more "physical" in character, focusing on architectural, rather than policy and program, variables. Specifically, the common theme of these five guidelines is the arrangement of spaces relative to one another to provide areas for specialized activities, define levels of privacy, or ensure views and use of the exterior.

The special characteristics of people with dementia necessitate building organization schemes that are particularly easy to understand and within which it is easy to find one's way. To maintain the homelike character of the environment, familiar spaces (e.g., outdoor planting areas, private bedrooms, semiprivate spaces for socializing) should be provided. These spaces must be situated to increase the environment's responsiveness to the specific needs of people with dementia (e.g., wandering paths should link major social spaces and should reinforce wandering as a meaningful activity; activity spaces should be clustered in a pattern similar to those in familiar single family homes). In addition, environments must reinforce the sense of dignity, privacy, and autonomy of people with dementia. For this reason, it is important to organize space to provide opportunities for private conversation and reflection, normal socializing, and the exercise of independent choice and decision making.

4.1 Clusters of Small Activity Spaces

The creation of small groupings of people with dementia is an important goal for both facility planning (see principle 2.3: Appropriate Group Size) and design. In facilities with large undifferentiated spaces accommodating many users, such group definition is difficult. The clustering of a number of smaller spaces supporting a range of related activities (e.g., cooking, dining, and doing laundry) can reinforce group identity.

People with Dementia

With their diminished ability to think and reason in complex ways, people with dementia experience increasing difficulty in perceiving and processing information about their environment. The transition from one's home to any group setting can thus be extremely stressful, as residents are likely to be overwhelmed by the complexity and unfamiliarity of the group setting (Peppard 1986). This may result in feelings of confusion, disorientation, and helplessness.

People with dementia might become further confused when they are ex-

Needs and Goals

People with Dementia

- *Decreased capabilities in perceiving and processing environmental information.*

- *Increased confusion in fulfilling normal, everyday tasks in unfamiliar environments.*

pected to carry out their normal patterns of behavior in a new environment to which they cannot relate. It is therefore important to create a social and physical environment that clearly helps them to identify their place within the whole. Creating small clusters of activities and spaces is a potentially effective way to orient people with dementia to their new environment. The social structure of groups should be supported through a physical organization of spaces that creates independent territories for individual or "household" use.

Therapeutic Goals

- *Maximize awareness and orientation with respect to time and place.*
- *Retain links with the healthy and familiar.*
- *Encourage increased social contact.*

Therapeutic Goals

Because dementia may engender confusion and disorientation with respect to time and place, program, policy, and design must all be aimed at maximizing the awareness and orientation of people with dementia to their physical and social environment. The goal is to help people with dementia redefine their social roles in new environments with clearly defined activities and spaces.

The creation of small clusters and their associations of home, together with activities of daily living, can serve to establish links with familiar experiences from the past. Moreover, consistent social contact with a limited number of people, often in the context of familiar activities, can foster greater social contact.

Design Concepts

Spatial Clusters

The strategy of clustering a number of smaller spaces may be utilized across a range of facilities for people with dementia. The core of each small area can establish a public zone surrounded by more private, specialized spaces (fig. 4.1). In long-term care facilities and group homes, one or more such residential clusters with living, dining, and cooking areas may be located at the center, surrounded by resident rooms. In some facilities, these groupings of resident rooms form "households" or "family clusters" (fig. 4.2). In day care settings, more specialized spaces, such as a beauty shop, quiet room, or kitchenette, might surround more public spaces (fig. 4.3).

Maximizing the Mix of Homelike Activities

In addition to the clustering of spaces, opportunities should be provided for a range of activities that come as close as possible to those typically found in homes. Some of these might include cooking and dining, games, and exercise. Organization or integration of these activities in much the same way as living room, dining room, and kitchen serve as the core in family homes can contribute to a higher degree of normalization (fig. 4.4). Additionally, the environment should allow clear identification of different activity areas, helping people with dementia to orient themselves to their new surroundings and enhancing legibility and familiarity.

Related Principles

Shared Spaces 5.2
Activity Alcoves 5.5

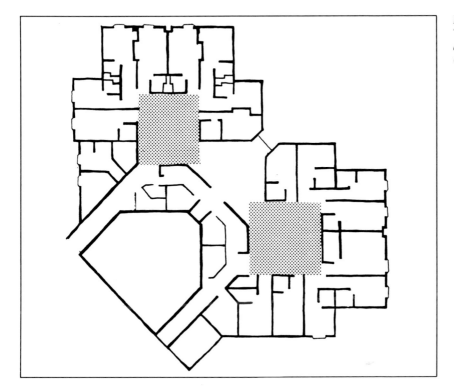

Figure 4.1
The butterfly plan provides communal areas adjacent to each cluster of twelve residents (Stevens 1987).

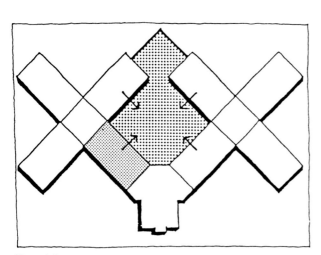 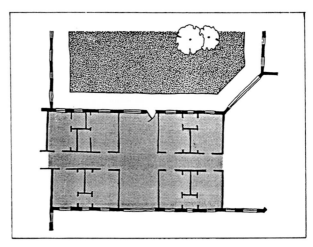

Figure 4.2
A "household" comprising a group of eight resident rooms, with a central, shared living/dining area at the center.

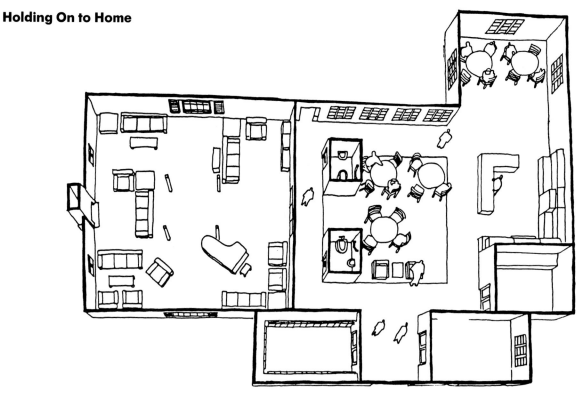

Figure 4.3
In this day care setting, the more specialized activities, including a barber shop, music area, and kitchenette, have been grouped around the more general sitting areas that occupy the core of the facility.

Figure 4.4
The public core of this facility comprises living, dining, lounge, kitchen, and pantry areas, organized in a way that is comparable to the core of most family homes.

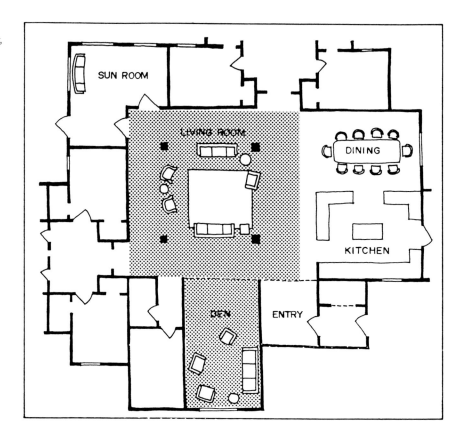

Wandering is a fairly common behavior of people with dementia. It should be viewed as an opportunity for meaningful activity, rather than only as a problem associated with this population. Both the physical and the organizational environment should be supportive of this activity, allowing it to occur in appropriate settings with well-defined and secure wandering paths.

4.2 Opportunities for Meaningful Wandering

People with Dementia

Wandering, for this population, can be defined as "extended periods of aimless or disoriented movement without full awareness of one's behavior" (Namazi, Rosner & Calkins 1989, 1). The three types of wandering most commonly found among people with dementia are (1) restless activity-seeking, typically found in environments that provide few opportunities to engage the residents; (2) habitual activity stemming from previous experiences; and (3) disorientation resulting from the inability to find one's way within a setting (Gilleard 1984). Wandering may be associated with other problematic behaviors that disrupt the unit routine or upset other clients; these include leaving the unit, rummaging in other residents' or staff's belongings, and verbally or physically threatening others (Namazi, Rosner & Calkins 1989).

Organizational Needs

Wandering is one of the most potentially difficult behaviors that face caregivers of people with dementia (Snyder et al. 1978). Wanderers may try to leave the facility and may easily become lost. Even within the facility, there is the possibility that residents will wander into unsafe areas where accidents may occur (e.g., outdoor ponds, staircases). Traditionally, facilities have dealt with wandering through the use of restraints, both physical and chemical. Increasingly, however, this has come to be regarded as inappropriate and even counter-productive. Ethically, the use of restraints is considered dehumanizing and in violation of client dignity. Restrained residents have also been shown to suffer from more falls than unrestrained residents (Green 1987). On a practical level, restrained patients require increased skin care and must be constantly repositioned, toileted, and hydrated, with consequent increases in nursing care and charting time (Namazi, Rosner & Calkins 1989).

It is important to recognize that wandering behavior need not necessarily have negative connotations. Coons (1988) pointed out, for example, that some authors refer to wandering paths as "racetracks." The negative architectural qualities of many settings for wandering behavior may be responsible for such unfavorable associations. A meaningful wandering path can begin to address those negative aspects, providing a positive outcome.

Therapeutic Goals

Wandering can serve as an outlet for a number of needs of people with dementia. It can provide residents with a degree of stimulation and challenge and can become a meaningful activity, rather than merely physical exercise.

Needs and Goals

People with Dementia

- *Some forms of wandering may be a response to limitations of the environment.*

Organizational Goal

- *Treat wandering behavior as an opportunity rather than as a problem, with responsive programs and an accommodating physical environment.*

Therapeutic Goals

- *Moderate stimulation and challenge.*

- *Maximize orientation to space and time.*
- *Ensure safety and security.*

The environment should have sufficient cues so that people with dementia do not resort to wandering as a consequence of disorientation (Hussian & Brown 1987). The goal is maximization of orientation and awareness of the physical environment at all times. To ensure both physical safety and psychological security of people with dementia, wandering paths should be free of potential dangers and yet provide more than the "racetrack" environment.

Design Concepts

Continuity

Continuity is one desirable characteristic for wandering paths. There is sufficient evidence to suggest that dead-end paths cause frustration and agitation. Therefore, design applications that incorporate some measure of continuity and form a continuous loop are preferable to dead-end or interrupted paths (figs. 4.5 and 4.6).

Figure 4.5
Here, continuity is provided by a path surrounding a large interior space. This path wraps around a public activity area, shares in the open feeling of the environment—unlike a restricted corridor—and still has its own definition, which is provided by the use of a darker floor material to designate the wandering area. (The Weiss Institute, Philadelphia Geriatric Center.)

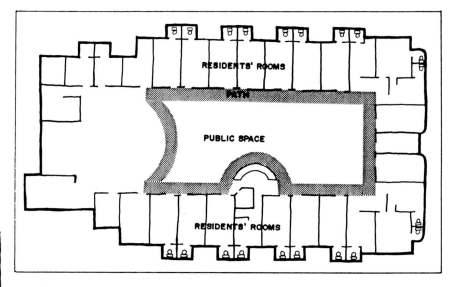

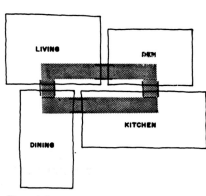

Figure 4.6
The concept of a "continuous loop" is not exclusive to large facilities. This schematic diagram illustrates the potential to accommodate a path in the context of a house or a group home by using interconnected spaces—kitchen, dining, living, and family rooms—that make up the public domain of the house. To form a path in a small single family house, it is often useful to arrange furniture against the walls and to remove coffee tables with dangerous sharp corners that might endanger the wanderer.

Understandable Paths

It is important that paths for wandering be legible and understandable to people with dementia. When paths are located out of doors, only one entrance or exit door should provide access to the path; residents may be disoriented and confused if they find themselves reentering the facility at a point different than that from which they left. Paths should be simple to comprehend whether they are indoors or outdoors (fig. 4.7). Wandering paths that are too long or complicated or cover too much territory will be disorienting and frustrating to wanderers, who may become "trapped" on the path if they cannot recognize a familiar exit point.

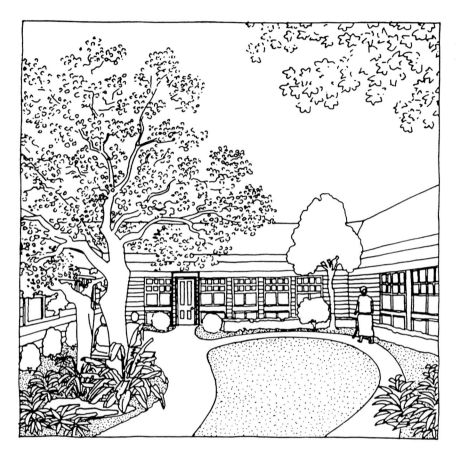

Figure 4.7
A prominent, unambiguous, single entry/exit point and a relatively short and simple path that can be viewed from every point make this wandering path negotiable and understandable.

Landmarks

While there is little research evidence that pertains specifically to wayfinding for people with dementia, it is reasonable to extrapolate from more general research on wayfinding among elderly persons in institutional settings (Weisman 1987). This research supports the hypothesis that the prevalence of repetitive modules can lead to wandering due to disorientation and an inability to find one's way in the environment. Introducing memorable and unique landmarks along the way can provide residents with cues for orientation (fig. 4.8). Landmarks need not be monumental in size or character; however, they should offer either a special meaning or a unique spatial identity.

Definition of Regions

While it is not clear whether color by itself can provide needed landmarks, it can certainly serve to enrich, enliven, and heighten stimulation in institutional environments. Color, types of furnishings, and finishes and materials can be developed around particular themes, thereby defining larger areas of a building as distinctive regions. To the extent that residents can recognize such regions (e.g., the several wings on a floor), these may serve to minimize prob-

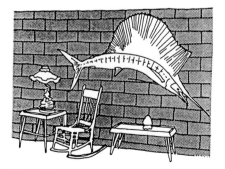

Figure 4.8
This unique personal object brought to the unit by a resident is displayed in the public circulation space, where it can assume the role of a "landmark"—a memorable orientational device.

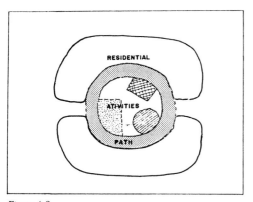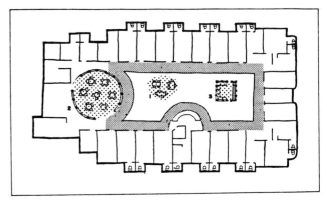

Figure 4.9
(a) This schematic drawing shows different zones within a large common area, surrounded by a wandering path. (b) This application of "defined regions" is located in a large unit: area 1 is a multipurpose space with tables and chairs, 2 is a dining area, and 3 is a gazebo. (The Weiss Institute, Philadelphia Geriatric Center.)

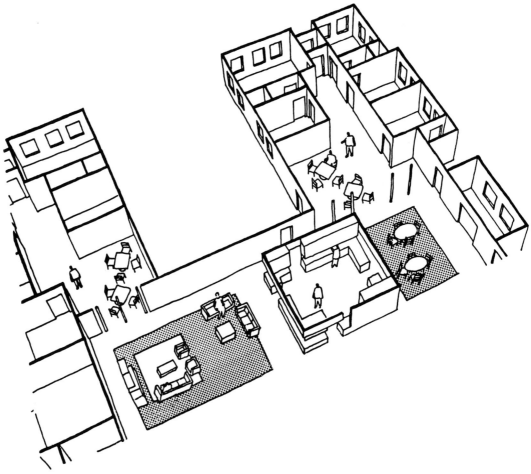

Figure 4.10
Each of the households faces the wandering path and a different activity area (e.g., dining, living). This functional differentiation helps in orientation.

lems of disorientation that can occur in large, visually undifferentiated institutional environments of repetitive modules (figs. 4.9 and 4.10).

Activity Alcoves

To ensure that wandering becomes more than just a meaningless physical activity, the wandering paths should provide elements of interest along the way. They can do so by having activity alcoves adjacent to, but not a part of, wandering paths, so that residents have the opportunity to participate without being required to do so (fig. 4.11).

Outdoor Paths

The outdoor loop is less restricted and can be spread over a considerable area without incurring excessive cost. Although the use of an outdoor path is limited in regions with inclement weather, creative use of the microclimate can extend the utility of the outdoors. Outdoor paths can introduce opportunities for activities and experiences that are not readily available indoors, such as walking through gardens or parklike spaces, stopping to look at or play with pets, or sunning outside at a bench along the path.

Positive Outdoor Spaces 4.3
Activity Alcoves 5.5

Related Principles

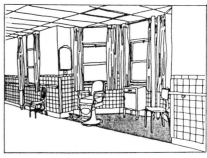

Figure 4.11
An activity alcove was developed here from an existing bay window area. The defined space is located adjacent to the wandering path, with visible activity—a barber shop. It provides a stopping place and a point of interest for wanderers.

Outdoor spaces provide unique and relatively less expensive settings that can meet a range of resident and client needs. Relief from the dominant ambience of the facility and appropriate stimulation for people with dementia can be provided here in different ways. These include thematic activities (e.g., gardening or caring for pets) and structured opportunities to observe naturally

4.3 Positive Outdoor Spaces

occurring events, such as seasonal changes and ongoing activities in the surroundings of interest to the residents. Positive outdoor spaces can provide variety in the life of people with dementia, offering a choice of familiar opportunities for socialization and privacy, for physical activities, and for contemplation within a safe, controlled environment. Providing views to the constantly changing outdoors can enhance residents' mood and orientation and serve to reduce the negative influence of the monolithic, institutional scale of larger facilities.

Needs and Goals

People with Dementia

- *Enclosed and nonstimulating environments can result in frustration and disruptive behavior.*

Therapeutic Goals

- *Regulate stimulation and challenge.*

- *Provide autonomy and control.*

- *Maintain awareness and orientation.*

- *Maintain ties to the healthy and familiar.*

- *Support functional ability through meaningful activity.*

People with Dementia

Oftentimes, people with dementia experience both temporal and spatial disorientation. They may be unable to distinguish day from night or to identify their present location (Gilleard 1984). Furthermore, confined, enclosed places are often unsettling for them (Laxton 1985). These problems are aggravated by the characteristics of traditional institutional settings, including long corridors lined with identical doors, the absence of windows, and generally very low levels of stimulation and contact with the outside world (Weisman 1987). The absence of family and of familiar environments and the inability to understand the reason for the change in their surroundings further exacerbate the fears and confusion of people with dementia.

Residents can benefit from a chance to release pent-up energy and frustration, particularly in settings that seem more familiar and comforting than the facility itself. The failure to provide such opportunities for the discharge of energy may precipitate disruptive behavior requiring the use of physical and chemical restraints.

Therapeutic Goals

It is important to recognize the need to provide people with dementia with regulated stimulation and challenge. Visual, olfactory, auditory, and tactile stimulation abound in nature. Outdoor spaces can provide residents with a wide range of manageable activities (e.g., gardening) that allow self-pacing and participation at different levels of skill and ability.

It is also important to provide people with dementia with opportunities for individual decision making, autonomy, and control. For this reason, outdoor spaces should have easy, independent access and should provide the individual with choices for contact and socializing, as well as for privacy and retreat.

The outdoor environment is essential in helping people with dementia to maintain clear perceptual links to familiar aspects of their spatial and temporal world. The "reality" of time of day or season of the year may be more effectively conveyed by a view to the outside environment that taps into long-term memory than by words alone. This may assist in increasing the residents' awareness of their surroundings and in exposing them to regulated degrees of stimulation by establishing visual links with the outside.

The outdoor environment is an excellent tool for enhancing a nonmedical, noninstitutional, positive facility image for people with dementia, staff, and family members. This image might help to encourage visits and volunteering and thus provide a better quality of life for residents. It has been suggested that attractive landscaping also promotes staff satisfaction and helps to reduce the rapid turnover endemic in long-term care facilities (Rapelje, Papp & Crawford, no date). Environments patterned after the outside community, with an emphasis on wellness, can help clients maintain ties with the healthy and familiar, presenting opportunities to integrate current experiences and relationships with the past.

Outdoor Opportunities

Outdoor spaces can offer unique opportunities for a wide range of stimulating activities—activities that might not be feasible or desirable in the indoor setting. Outdoor spaces offer different opportunities for exercise (e.g., ambulatory residents can engage in shuffleboard, croquet, bocci ball), socializing, and a breath of fresh air. When the weather permits, the outdoors is an alternative to the dayroom for many group activities and planned special events, such as barbecues, birthdays, and holiday celebrations. Raised planting beds that are wheelchair-accessible can provide residents with the opportunity to engage in gardening. Water features located in well-landscaped outdoor spaces offer visual, tactile, and auditory stimulation. Outdoor alcoves will give residents secluded places in which to visit with family members or from which to observe outdoor activities. Delightful paths for wandering can be created—negotiable and comprehensible paths that circle gardens and pass by places for sitting. Provision of outdoor washroom facilities is an added bonus.

Care should be taken to extend the noninstitutional image and scale of the facility to the outdoors through such devices as small groupings of familiar outdoor furnishings and provisions for pets, birdfeeders, etc. (figs. 4.12 to 4.14).

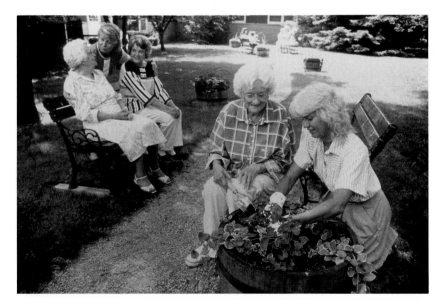

Design Concepts

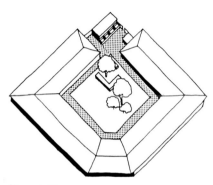

Figure 4.12
The enclosed courtyard includes seating, raised planters, and a grassy area surrounded by a paved path. The corner structure is a "mini-zoo," with several animals cared for jointly by residents and staff. (The Cedar Lake Home Tri-Campus, West Bend, Wis.).

Figure 4.13
The paved part of the green courtyard provides a path for wandering, as well as a platform for flexible backyard seating that is quite domestic. The implied control of social grouping and communication, the provision for exercising choice in group size and location, and the beautiful landscaping all convey a positive, noninstitutional image. (Courtesy of Susan Larson, New Perspectives, Wis.; photographed by David C. Denemark.)

Figure 4.14
In certain locations, such as in this Florida day care setting, the outdoor space is a viable part-time alternative to indoor spaces for most of the year.

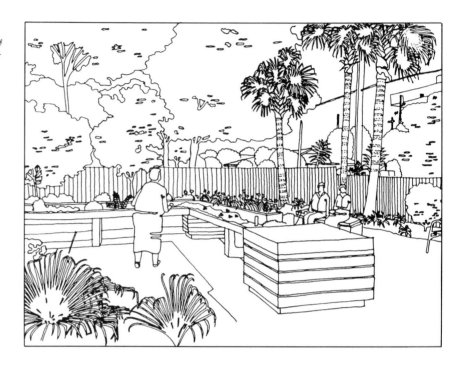

Figure 4.14
In certain locations, such as in this Florida day care setting, the outdoor space is a viable part-time alternative to indoor spaces for most of the year.

The latter might also act as stimulus for conversation; in addition, caring for pets may give residents a sense of responsibility and a chance to display affection. (See design principles: 4.2 Opportunities for Meaningful Wandering, 4.4 Other Living Things, 5.5 Activity Alcoves, and 3.1 Noninstitutional Character.)

A View to the Outside

Views to outdoor areas can be just as important as the provision of usable outdoor spaces. Such views will increase resident orientation to time, space, and season and will ensure a less institutional image for the facility. Views from resident rooms are usually mandated by law, but residents also spend a great deal of time in public spaces such as lounges and lobbies, where views are not required. Outdoor views from public areas will reduce the sense of confinement and provide valuable stimuli and information to clients. Views to the outdoors along staircases and in corridors and elevator lobbies serve to minimize the traditional "institutional" image and provide increased levels of sensory input in public areas (fig. 4.15). These views will be especially effective if they are located at key decision-making points and if they lead to accessible outdoor areas. Skylights can also be used to admit light and provide a link with the outside where other types of views may not be possible (fig. 4.16).

In some instances, views to the outside may be considered undesirable, as when views are provided from places that house activities requiring residents' undivided attention. For example, some facility managers and staff members suggest that outdoor views from dining rooms may distract residents from eating, although there is no general consensus as to whether this is true.

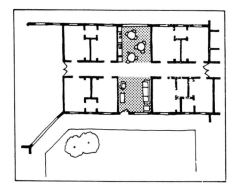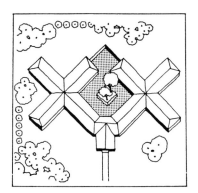

Figure 4.15
(a) The eight room unit illustrated has public spaces—dining and living rooms—at the center of the unit. This interruption in the conventional double-loaded corridor provides a break in the potential monotony of the circulation path.
(b) The windows on both sides of all units overlook the courtyard on one side and a distant pastoral landscape on the other. (The Cedar Lake Home Tri-Campus, West Bend, Wis.)

Unobtrusive Enclosure and Physical Safety

The outdoor space should be simple and safe from physical and perceptual obstacles to movement and ambulation. All plants and materials used in outdoor spaces should be nontoxic. Attention should be paid to the nature of the enclosure; unlike functional chain link fences, boundaries defined by plants or the configuration of the building mass are typically unobtrusive and have the same potential effectiveness (fig. 4.17).

Unobtrusive Observation

Outdoor enclosures should allow easy, efficient staff observation that is not disturbingly obvious to the resident. Residents will appreciate free access to

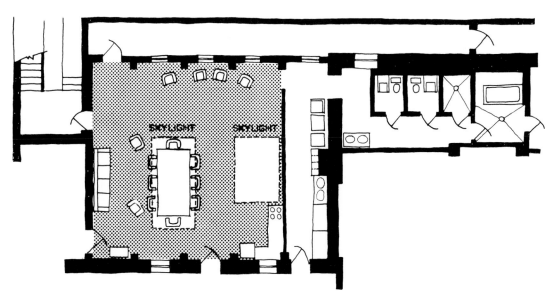

Figure 4.16
In facilities such as this day care center, where public areas are totally or partially enclosed in the interior of the building, skylights can admit light and provide a link with the outside. In addition to admitting daylight, the skylight can define and differentiate activity zones, such as the dining or kitchen area. (St. Ann's Day Care Center; St. Francis, Wisconsin.)

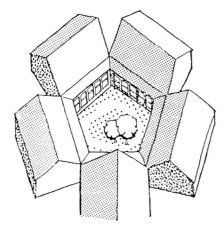

Figure 4.17
In this "star plan," the outdoor courtyard is physically and visually accessible from the households of the most active residents. The perimeter of the courtyard is a continuous wandering path within a micro-climate that can extend the use of the space. The grassy courtyard is a potential space for many activities, from gardening to passive sitting. Being surrounded by four residential wings, the space requires no obtrusive barriers for safety and control.

outdoor spaces without the need for staff permission or constant supervision. The need for easy surveillance of all residents from central points where staff members can observe most residents (and still perform other tasks) necessitates a wide field of vision without major visual obstacles (fig. 4.18).

Positive Microclimate

People with dementia are likely to be aged and therefore more sensitive to harsh weather conditions, from which they must be protected. The creation of a positive microclimate for this population calls for warm southern exposures and protection from wind and excessive sun. Effective design features, such as strategically placed planting to act as wind breaks, trees to provide shade, and the building mass itself for enclosure, can extend the time and season of use of outdoor spaces (fig. 4.19).

Flexible Seating

The type of seating provided is a major determinant of whether an outdoor space will be successful. Whyte (1980) emphasized that people appreciate an opportunity to arrange their seating so as to provide maximum social comfort and privacy, to take greatest advantage of sunlight and windblocks, and to situate themselves where there is a view to ongoing activity. In some instances, the opportunity to arrange seating for privacy and comfort may be more significant than whether or not people actually do so. For these reasons, flexible, movable seating should be provided whenever possible. In addition,

Figure 4.18
To provide an uninterrupted view across the courtyard, low shrubs and trees with canopies above eight feet are used.

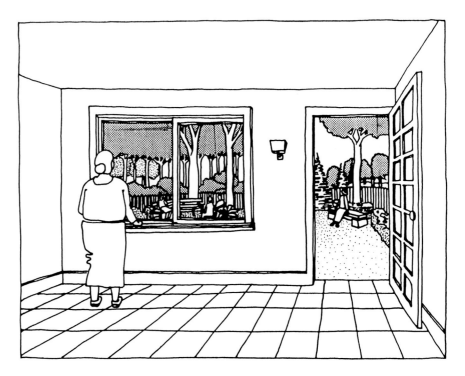

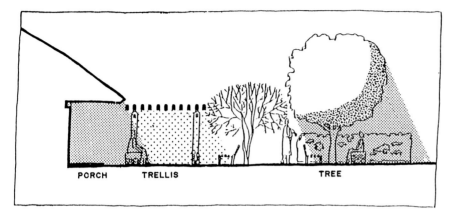

Figure 4.19
The introduction of degrees of shelter—from sun, rain, and wind—can extend the use of this outdoor area by providing varying levels of climatic protection suited to individual needs.

PORCH   TRELLIS   TREE

seating of various types should be provided in many different locations within the outdoor space: near entry and exit doors, near planned activity nodes (e.g., close to gardening beds), near ongoing daily activities (so that residents can watch the lawn being mowed, flowers being watered, etc.), in tranquil and private sections, and on the route of travel within the area (e.g., at various points along the wandering path) (Regnier 1985).

In planning seating for outdoor areas, there are many possible activities that should be accommodated, including both spontaneous encounters and spontaneous observation of nature and staff, neighborhood, and other residents' activities and planned activities (e.g., musical events, puppet shows). There should be space to accommodate wheelchair users for these activities. Characteristics of successful seating arrangements include variety, flexibility, social comfort (i.e., seating arrangements should not force eye contact or social interaction), and consideration of weather extremes (i.e., seating should be placed to avoid harsh sunlight or wind). Appropriate types of seating are comfortable (the majority of the seats should have backs and arms to aid residents in sitting down and getting up), anthropometrically correct for elderly persons, lightweight (so that they can be easily rearranged by either residents or staff), double-functioning (e.g., a ledge around one side of a raised planting bed might also function as a bench), and esthetically pleasing (stereotypic "institutional" choices should be avoided) (Regnier 1985) (fig. 4.20).

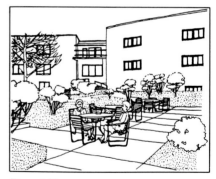

Figure 4.20
Sturdy, vinyl-coated metal chairs and matching tables are one of the seating arrangements appropriate for outdoor use.

4.4 Other Living Things

Environments for people with dementia can be greatly enriched through the incorporation of plants and animals. Flowers, greenhouses, birdfeeders, mini-zoos, and household pets all are potential means of increasing residents' interaction with other living things.

People with Dementia

Central to human behavior are the activities that revolve around responsibilities to other living entities, their nurturance, and maintenance. This in-

Needs and Goals

People with Dementia

- *Assuming even limited responsibility for living things can increase feelings of autonomy and control among people with dementia.*

- *Living things can be used to enhance sensory stimulation and add variety to the of activities of people with dementia.*

Therapeutic Goals

- *Maximize autonomy and control.*

- *Establish links to the healthy and familiar.*

- *Provide opportunities for social interaction.*

- *Provide opportunities for stimulation and challenge.*

Concepts for Planning and Design

terdependence among living things fosters a sense of pride, as people observe changes for which they can take some credit. People with dementia, however, may often find themselves cast into the role of a "dependent," unable to continue to care for their families or themselves. Incorporating living things, including pets, plants, and other people, into the environments of people with dementia can act as a compensatory measure.

An empirical study by Langer and Rodin (1976) explored the effects of enhanced personal responsibility and choice on nursing home residents. Residents in the experimental group were offered the opportunity to keep and care for a plant. Those in the control group were given plants and told that the nurses would look after these. A statistically significant improvement on measures of alertness, active participation, and sense of general well-being was reported for the experimental group.

Pet therapy and the benefits associated with caring for pets is another new and exciting area of exploration that holds promise for application in environments for people with dementia. Anecdotal evidence supporting the use of pets was reported by Rapelje, Papp, and Crawford (1981). Influenced by a positive experience in another nursing home where a resident was permitted to bring his dog, the Home for Senior Citizens in Welland, Ontario, is planning to purchase a dog that will be cared for and housed on the premises. The presence of a familiar pet is expected to provide stimulation, affection, and companionship for the residents.

Therapeutic Goals

The addition of living things to environments for people with dementia can be used to reinforce feelings of control, especially when residents assume primary responsibility for the care of plants or pets. Living things can also add a noninstitutional dimension of healthy familiarity to the environment, reinforcing its domestic nature. In this instance, a minor addition to the setting (e.g., the institution of a small greenhouse area for plants within an Alzheimer's unit) may have a significant positive influence on residents' perception of the environment.

Related to design principle 3.3 Things from the Past, living things can contribute to reminiscence, which may foster social interaction between residents and staff or visitors. Residents can benefit from the changing stimulation provided by the growth of plants: their odors, colors, flowers, and shapes. Pets also provide varying visual and auditory stimulation.

Greenhouses, Sun Rooms, and Places for Plants

Residents' enjoyment of flowers and other plants need not be restricted to a gardening area or outdoor courtyard. Special areas might be set aside to enjoy nature indoors through the creation of a "greenhouse" or designated "natural" area within the facility (fig. 4.21). Such places can be conceptualized as ranging along a continuum of scale from a major outdoor space to a greenhouse (similar to those attached to some single-family homes), a sun room or a symbolic "plant" area created out of a small nook or alcove, or small, discrete areas

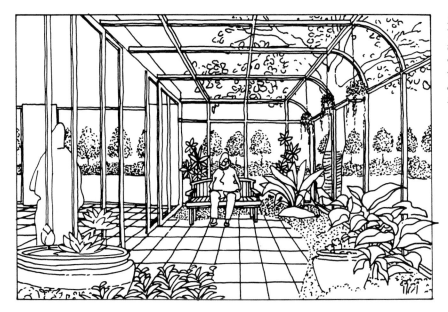

Figure 4.21
The creation of a greenhouse is one strategy for incorporating plants into facilities for people with dementia. These increase the residential nature of the facility and at the same time serve as a source of visual, tactile, and olfactory stimulation.

for plants throughout the facility (even including residents' rooms). All of these locations can serve the similar function of improving the quality of life for people with dementia.

Plants can be incorporated into the environment as an attractive form of sensory stimuli. The greenhouse or area for plants might be filled year-round with seasonal flowers, easy-to-grow vegetables, and other varied and attractive plants, all providing a source of visual, olfactory, and tactile stimulation for residents.

Caring for plants is a meaningful activity for which residents can assume responsibility. Each might be allowed to take a plant for his or her room. The greenhouse area might be designed to accommodate a few seats as well, thereby creating a quiet place for solitude and a nook for visiting with family and friends. Flowers from the greenhouse can serve as centerpieces for special meals and provide bouquets for residents' birthdays. In these ways, the creation of a greenhouse enhances the noninstitutional image of the facility, making it more pleasant for residents, visitors, and staff.

As a necessary precaution, all plants in facilities for people with dementia should be nontoxic.

Household Pets

The ways in which pets can be introduced into a facility are varied, and caregivers should select the particular options that are most appropriate for their situation. A facility might explore the therapeutic potential of pets without a large initial commitment through participation in a visiting pets program, in which volunteers from a local humane society bring animals to visit nursing home residents on a regular basis. Adoption of a pet, such as a cat or dog, by each household is another method for building a sense of community or family within the facility (fig. 4.22). Such a pet should be even-tempered and affec-

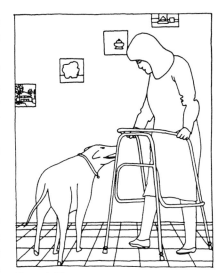

Figure 4.22
The use of pets in facilities for people with dementia serves as a stimulus to conversation (e.g., with visiting relatives), activities (e.g., grooming, walking, feeding), and companionship.

tionate—a local pet shop can offer valuable advice on choosing an animal—and caregivers should check the allergy history of residents before proceeding with this suggestion. Some facilities have gone so far as to incorporate a "mini-zoo" into their outdoor area, including such animals as rabbits and baby goats or sheep.

Where particular types of adaptations (e.g., an outdoor mini-zoo) are disallowed due to policy mandates or regulatory standards, a singing or talking bird is a cheerful addition to a reception area or lounge; bird feeders located adjacent to windows where they are visible to residents may have many of the same benefits. A tank of colorful tropical fish can provide a point of interest in a day room or activity area; watching a tank of fish is reported to have a calming effect on many people. Finally, caring for and playing with pets provide additional activities or "something to do" with visiting family and friends. Facilities for people with dementia should avail themselves of as many of these opportunities as possible.

Related Principles	Positive Outdoor Spaces 4.3

4.5 Public to Private Realms

People with dementia should be allowed to choose from a variety of public to private spaces. This continuum of public to private realms, created through both physical design and organizational policy, facilitates individual control of sensory stimulation, social interaction, and involvement in activities.

Needs and Goals

People with Dementia

• *Residents may have strong reactions to perceived intrusion of personal space and infringement on independence.*

People with Dementia

Few facilities for people with dementia provide a continuum of public to private spaces. Group homes and long-term care facilities most often accommodate their residents in double occupancy rooms. Day care centers rarely have private spaces to which users can retreat. Small group activities, such as visiting with family or friends, often must take place in public lounges and even in corridors. Organizational policy may likewise compromise opportunities for privacy within the environment (e.g., opening closed doors without knocking compromises residents' privacy even within their own rooms).

People with dementia are highly sensitive to environmental stimulation and may become overstressed or anxious if exposed to stimulation that is beyond their already lowered tolerance level. They often react strongly to what they perceive as threatening intrusions to personal space and independence. Many of the problem behaviors associated with dementia are influenced by environmental factors. Greater choice and control in the environment, with respect to sensory stimulation, social interaction, and involvement in activities, can reduce the frequency and intensity of these behaviors.

Organizational Needs

Facilities that provide care for people with dementia must ensure their physical safety and security; this is often accomplished through constant supervision and surveillance. However, policies that prohibit spending time alone in one's room may compromise privacy and control by people with dementia. Likewise, the physical design of spaces without defined boundaries can compromise the need for privacy.

Therapeutic Goals

People with dementia should be able to engage in social behavior at a number of different levels, from active engagement with others to passive involvement through observation. Forced sharing of a space may actually inhibit rather than facilitate social contact. In the absence of physical privacy, people may withdraw from others as a means of obtaining psychological privacy (DeLong 1970).

People with dementia should be provided with regulated stimulation and challenge and not be forced to deal with degrees of stimulation beyond their tolerance level at a given time. The domestic environments that people typically occupy throughout their lives support a range of public and private behaviors. To the extent possible, environments for people with dementia should provide this same range of opportunities (fig. 4.23).

Therapeutic Goals

- *Allow opportunities for privacy.*
- *Regulate stimulation and challenge.*
- *Provide opportunities for social contact.*

The spaces within a home were characterized by Alexander, Ishikawa and Silverstein (1977) as falling along an "intimacy gradient," reflecting the level of privacy/openness of each. The following concepts reflect the characteristics of space and activities at four points along this gradient.

Design Concepts

Spaces for Solitude

While acknowledging concerns of safety, security, and staff surveillance, spaces should be included where people with dementia can sometimes be by themselves. In some facilities, private resident rooms would provide the necessary solitude. Where this is not possible, however, there should be defined spaces—sufficiently small, soft, and comfortable—that respond to the need for solitude and quiet contemplation (fig. 4.24).

Protected Spaces

There are occasions when a small group—people with dementia, caregivers, family, or friends—may want to be together in a space protected from unwanted sensory stimulation and social encroachment. This level of protection can be achieved either by increasing physical distance from major activity/traffic zones or by enhancing the sense of enclosure and spatial definition of these spaces (figs. 4.25 and 4.26). Furniture arrangement in these spaces should be sociopetal—encouraging social interaction—to facilitate better social contact.

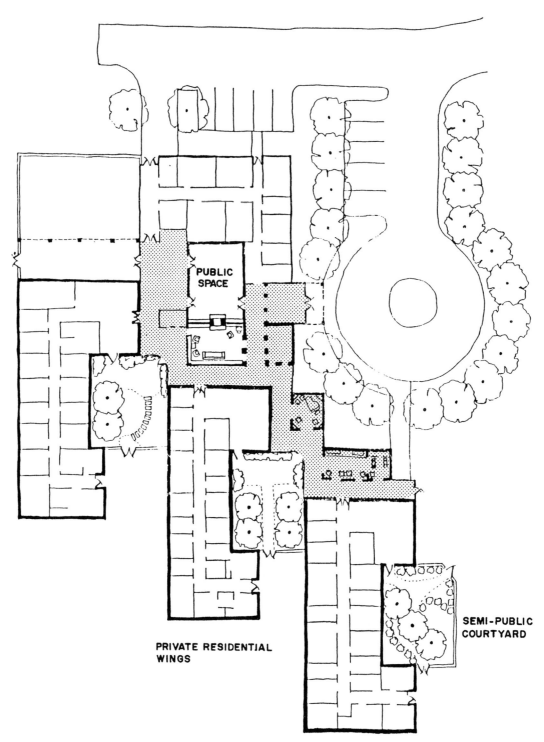

Figure 4.23
This plan of a facility for people with dementia includes a variety of spaces ranging from public (living room, kitchen, garden) to private (quiet alcove, private room). (Woodside Place, Oakmont, Pa.; Perkins, Geddes, Eastman, Architects.)

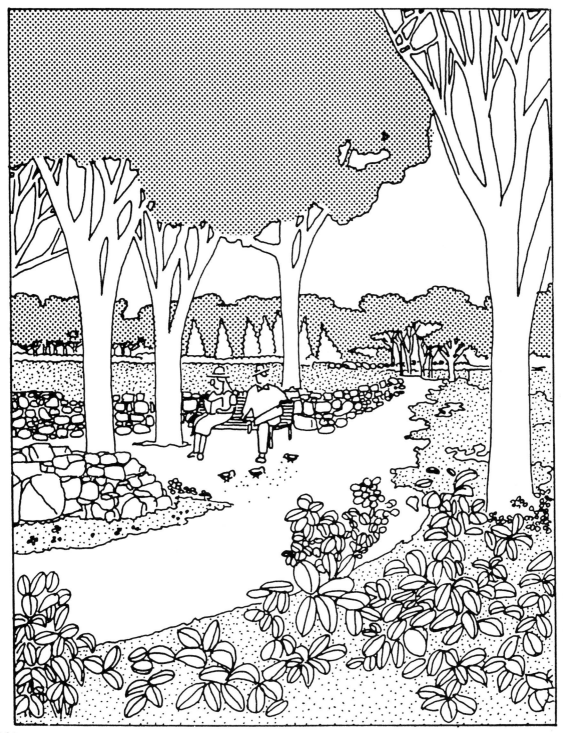

Figure 4.24
This area for quiet contemplation has been created out-of-doors in a clearing surrounded by trees, off of a path. The bench and the setting ensure solitude and support small group gatherings of not more than two to three people.

Figure 4.25
A semiprivate area can serve as an appealing
shared social space for small groups and for
visiting with family and friends.

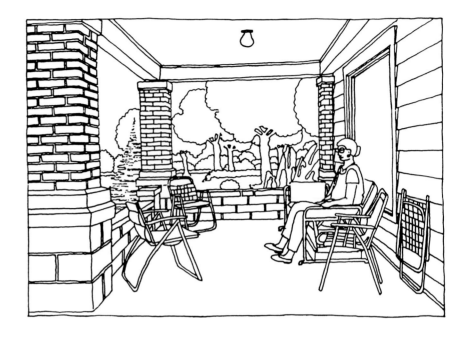

Figure 4.26
A comfortably furnished "nook" can function as
a semiprivate space for small group conversa-
tions or just for sitting.

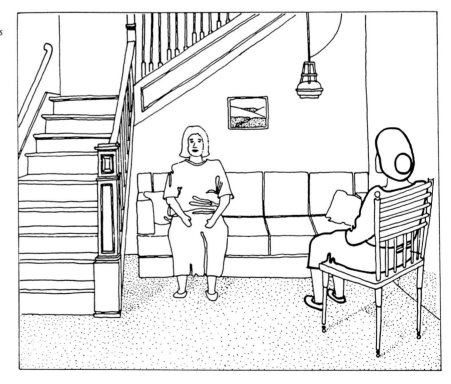

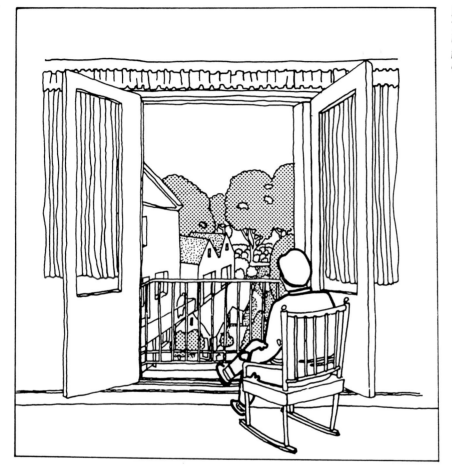

Figure 4.27
This arrangement—a set of doors leading to a balcony—can function as an effective front porch, providing views to people and ongoing activities.

In-between Spaces

Spaces adjacent to, but not a part of, activity zones can provide a "front porch" that allows passive observation without the necessity of active participation in ongoing activities (figs. 4.27 to 4.29). These intermediate spaces provide opportunities to "preview" (Zeisel, Welch & Demos 1978) activities without a commitment to involvement or participation.

Public Spaces

Finally, at the public end of the continuum, are spaces to which all people have equal and unimpeded access. Such spaces can include lobbies, activity rooms, and congregate dining facilities. These spaces are important activity areas for those residents who are able to deal with higher levels of stimulation. However, not all people will want to use these spaces, and no one will want to use them all of the time.

Given the great numbers of people and the potential for high levels of stimulation, the design of these spaces should ensure that people with dementia

Figure 4.28
A window seat adjacent to a circulation path can serve as a place for gathering or just passive observation of activities.

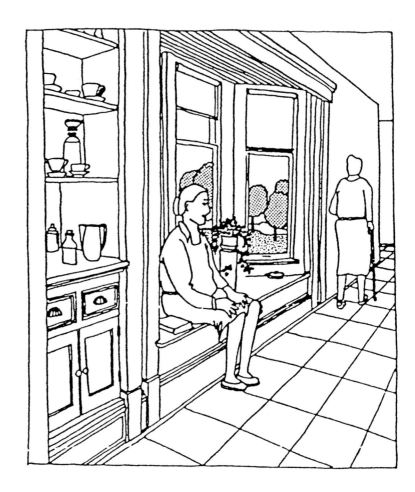

Figure 4.29
Defined activity areas separated from major paths of circulation provide semiprivate areas. (The Washington Home, Washington, D.C.; Dudens and Knoop, Architects.)

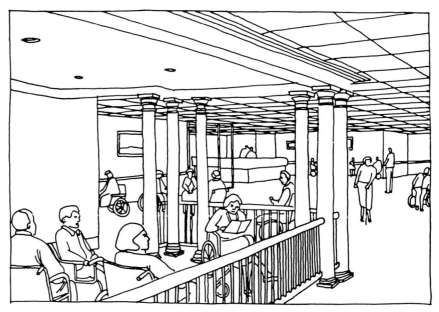

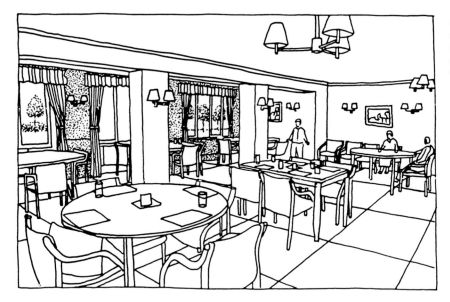

Figure 4.30
Spatial differentiation through the use of col-
umns, small groups of tables, and various levels
of lighting serves to make this congregate dining
room manageable for people with dementia.

are not overwhelmed either visually or socially. This can be done through spatial differentiation (fig. 4.30), dampening extraneous stimuli through acoustical design, and use of appropriate scale.

Intimate Dining 5.4
Activity Alcoves 5.5
Resident Rooms 5.6

Related Principles

Overleaf: Jerry Schmidt, photographed by Susie Post

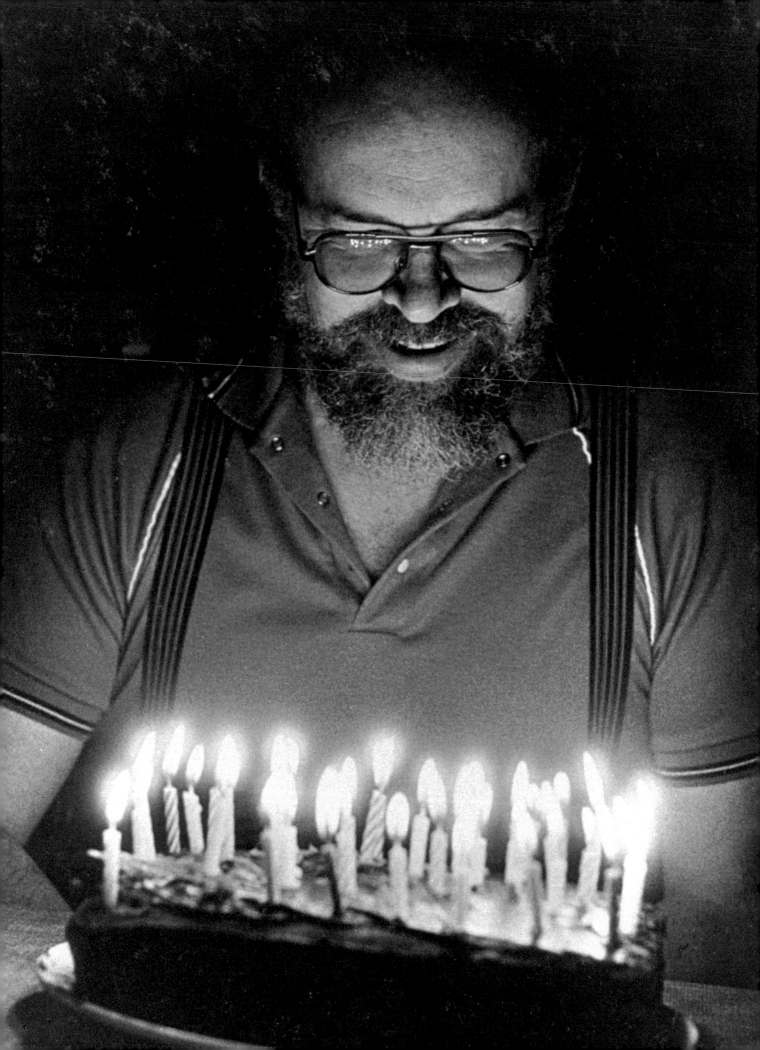

5 Principles for Design: Activity Areas

This final set of design principles focuses on specific spaces for particular activities or events. Recommendations are made for the types of activities that must be accommodated, for the characteristics that these spaces should embody, and for the therapeutic and organizational goals that should be supported through the design of such spaces. For example, design principle 5.3 recommends that kitchen facilities be provided for use by residents in facilities for people with dementia; these kitchens might be used by residents to independently carry on familiar and healthy activities, such as doing dishes, making a cup of coffee, or chatting over a kitchen table. To meet the needs of people with dementia for autonomy and control, maintenance of links with their past, and opportunities for socialization, kitchen spaces for use by residents should be residential in character and scale, a quality that might be achieved through the use of domestic furnishings and finishes (e.g., curtains in the window, a tablecloth on the wooden table for four people, and pictures and a calendar on the wall). These domestic kitchen spaces can also be designed to fulfill the organizational need for opportunities for unobtrusive observation of residents, which could be easily met through the provision of a kitchen "island" in the space, serving as an informal vantage point for staff members.

5.1 Entry and Transition

The entry sequence represents one's initial introduction to a facility for people with dementia. Entry design will be especially critical in facilities that experience a great deal of coming and going, such as day care and respite centers. A safe, protected, accessible entranceway should provide opportunities for unobtrusive monitoring of entering and exiting, appropriate space for storage of outerwear, and a comforting environment for leave-taking of people with dementia. Successful entry and transition areas should also provide an overview of the organization and general layout of the facility and a preview of ongoing activities, to aid in wayfinding and orientation for residents, staff members, and family caregivers.

People with Dementia

People with dementia often suffer from related problems (e.g., impaired mobility) that mandate special adaptations to make accessible means of entry and circulation in a facility or home. Problems of confusion and disorientation common among people with dementia may be exacerbated in unfamiliar set-

Needs and Goals

People with Dementia

- *May require special adaptations for accessibility and safe entry.*

- *Often disoriented in unfamiliar surroundings.*
- *Often have a distorted perception of depth.*

tings, especially when these are not the primary, residential setting with which the person is most familiar. (Such is the case with respite care, where the person only visits the setting occasionally.) Because of a distorted perception of depth (symptomatic of the disease), people with dementia may be further confused by seemingly ordinary, nonproblematic characteristics of entry and transition areas (e.g., strips of tape applied to the floor to increase traction may be perceived as a physical barrier) (Namazi, Rosner & Calkins 1989).

Caregivers' and Organizational Needs

- *Visiting an "Alzheimer's" facility may be distressing.*
- *Unobtrusive monitoring and control of the means of entry and exit are critical.*

Needs of Caregivers

Like people with dementia, family members and visiting friends can easily be threatened or put off by an "institutional" facility. They may be encouraged to visit if they experience the environment as familiar and supportive.

Organizational Needs

Organizations are very much aware of the need to monitor entry and access from Alzheimer's units and from the facility to the outside to prevent people with dementia from wandering away from designated areas or away from the facility. For this reason, it is important to provide means to control and supervise entry areas and circulation paths.

Therapeutic Goals

- *Ensure safety and security.*
- *Maximize awareness and orientation to place and time.*
- *Emphasize the healthy and familiar.*

Therapeutic Goals

Dementia may engender confusion and disorientation with respect to the physical environment. To maximize awareness and orientation of people with dementia to their physical surroundings, linkages between interior and exterior environments should be as clear and direct as possible. To the extent that a facility establishes linkages to the healthy and familiar (particularly to the residential), it can ease the discomfort of people with dementia and of their families and visitors.

Finally, to ensure the physical safety and psychological security of people with dementia, supervision of the transition area from the entry to the outside is required to prevent wandering away from the facility or into potentially dangerous areas. The transition from the entry to the core areas of the facility must ensure that the facility is physically accessible. Residents should not be expected to negotiate changes of level or confusing sequences of corridors or elevators, which may compound their sense of confusion and disorientation.

Design Concepts

Friendly Entrance

The entrance area greatly contributes to the first impression that both caregivers and people with dementia will have of the facility. For this reason, it is critical that the transition area—the place to take off coats, store things, and decide where to go next—and the entry be nonthreatening and welcoming. The entrance area should exude a comforting feeling to help alleviate anxiety about separation. Although it should be easily identifiable, there is no need for the entrance to be monumental in either size or scale. Domestic features

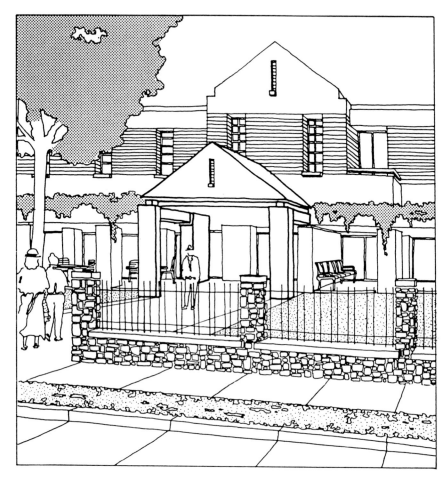

Figure 5.1
A separate entrance to a day care center in a long-term care building and the use of domestic architectural and landscaping features help to create a friendly, welcoming entry experience.

such as elements of a porch, lampposts, and shutters make the entrance area welcoming and friendly without becoming overwhelming for people with dementia (fig. 5.1). If a sign is necessary or desired, it should also be unobtrusive and should reinforce the image of a friendly entrance.

Sheltered and Accessible Entry

At the most basic level, entries into homes and facilities for people with dementia must be physically accessible. This may require the replacement of stairs with ramps (fig. 5.2), the enlargement of doorways to accommodate wheelchairs, and other related modifications. The entry into the facility should be at the same level and direct. Entryways should be sheltered from inclement weather (fig. 5.3), particularly in settings such as day care centers, where there is fairly constant movement of clients in and out of the building; caregivers will appreciate this amenity as well. The path from the drop-off point to the door should be short and safe and not require the person with dementia to encounter traffic or to make difficult decisions while entering

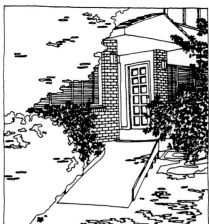

Figure 5.2
An inexpensive wood ramp was one of the few modifications needed to make this house accessible to a wheelchair user.

Figure 5.3
A drop-off point near the entrance to a day care center and an entrance sheltered from the elements make coming and going a protected and comfortable experience.

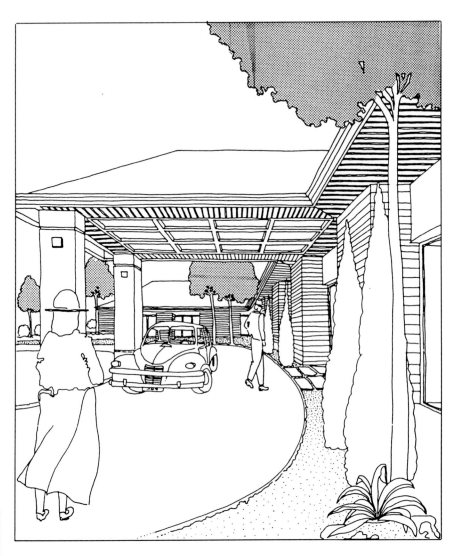

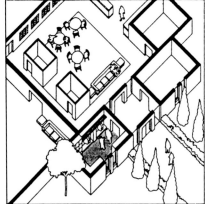

Figure 5.4
The entryway to this day care center has a walk-in closet room for storage and dressing that is near but visually sheltered from the main activity space.

or exiting the facility. It is possible to design for accessibility and still ensure that modifications look like integral parts of the home or facility and not just "add-ons."

Convenient Transition Area

Particularly in day care and respite centers, there is a need for a place adjacent to the means of entry that can serve as a transition area into the facility. This area should be welcoming and homelike to ease the apprehensions of confused clients and nervous or reluctant caregivers dropping off people with dementia. There should be provisions for storage, especially for coats and outer gear. Storage areas should be designed so that they are not readily apparent from the areas used by people with dementia (fig. 5.4), who may become preoccupied with rummaging in the closets or constantly putting on coats, hats, etc., in anticipation of the caregiver's return. A restroom located nearby will further enhance the convenience and efficiency of this space. The transition area itself should also be visually sheltered from the view of people in the public or activity areas of the facility, who may become distracted by constant activity near the entry.

Visible Destinations

To improve orientation and legibility, the transition area should either lead to or allow views to the interior spaces, so that people with dementia and visitors are able to see and understand the physical organization of the facility (fig. 5.5). A commanding vista of the entire facility is much preferred to the restricted view from a long, convoluted corridor for allowing one to understand the organization or plan of the building. For the same reason, the path from the outside of the facility to the destination should be as short and direct as possible. Landmarks can be used to reinforce the path to a destination that is not readily apparent.

Unobtrusive Vantage Point

It is of paramount importance that the entry and exit from the facility or home be supervised by staff to prevent people with dementia from wandering away. This can be accomplished through a variety of means, including mechanical or electronic devices, such as alarm systems and voice-controlled doors; a well-positioned administrative office or reception desk, with a door open to allow visual surveillance of the entry (fig. 5.6); or a caregiver who can be centrally positioned to monitor the door(s) into the unit. Many times, unobtrusive environmental solutions are less expensive and more sensitive to the needs of people with dementia than comparable "high-tech" solutions.

For the same reason, the door into a facility or household should be screened out as much as possible so as not to act as an enticement to the resident. This has been accomplished by painting doors the same color as the surrounding surfaces or by placing a piece of cloth over the push handle of an exit door to disguise it (Namazi, Rosner & Calkins 1989).

Noninstitutional Character 3.1

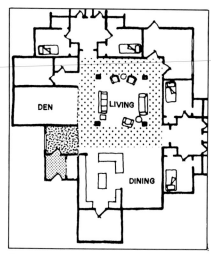

Figure 5.5
The organization of the floor plan of this small group home allows a person in the entry zone a clear view of the public areas of the home.

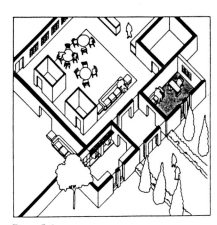

Figure 5.6
One alternative, sensitive method of providing unobtrusive control of the entry zone in a large facility is to place the administrative component —an office—with a staff member facing the transition area.

Related Principles

5.2 Shared Spaces

Many institutional settings for people with dementia are characterized by "null behavior" (Lawton 1981), a countertherapeutic condition of complete passivity. Shared spaces (Howell 1980) with scale and ambience comparable to that found at home can support opportunities for initiating activities, promote social contact, provide clients and residents with appropriate degrees of stimulation, and reinforce group identity.

Needs and Goals

People with Dementia

- *Residents appreciate and can benefit from moderated opportunities for socialization with others.*

Therapeutic Goals

- *Regulate stimulation.*
- *Create opportunities for increased social contact.*

Design Concepts

People with Dementia

While it is true that people with dementia may not be able to process high levels of stimulation or take on complex and demanding tasks without experiencing overload and distress, they still require opportunities to exercise remaining capabilities. In the absence of such opportunities capabilities may diminish even more rapidly (Lawton 1981).

Research in long-term care facilities suggests that interactions involving a large number of residents can result in stimulation overload; this in turn may cause ripples of negative behavior to spread over the whole group. Conversely, in situations where there are too few people, the variety of behaviors required for sufficient stimulation is not present; this represents null behavior (Lawton 1981).

Therapeutic Goals

Following Lawton's Theory of Adaptation and Aging, people with dementia should be provided with regulated levels of stimulation and appropriate challenge. The goal is one of exercising, but not overtaxing, remaining capabilities. Similarly, people with dementia should maximize opportunities that engage their social capabilities through interaction with peers, caregivers, families, and friends.

Facilities serving small populations (e.g., community group homes) will probably have smaller shared spaces. Some settings (e.g., long-term care facilities) may already have large shared spaces, such as a traditional day room, or may choose to develop such large spaces for group activities, such as dining. The following principles for design can minimize the problems of large spaces as well as maximize the potential of smaller shared spaces.

Figure 5.7
Each of the living units in this large group home is organized around a single open space that accommodates the living, dining, and kitchen areas. (Corrine Dolan Center, Heather Hill, Chardon, Ohio; Stephen Nemtin, Architect.)

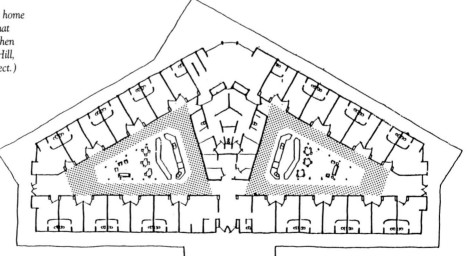

Small-Scale and Domestic Ambience

Large-scale institutional day rooms, often with extensive side-by-side seating along the wall (Sommer 1969) are not conducive to activities or social contact. As a consequence, activities are often displaced to corridors, a location that is neither desirable nor safe. Shared spaces, particularly those that must accommodate large numbers of people, should be subdivided into clearly identifiable activity areas of domestic scale (fig. 5.7). Such subdivision of space also responds to the need of people with dementia for privacy and passive participation.

The ambience of shared spaces should complement their domestic scale and residential qualities. Such ambience is in part a consequence of domestic materials and finishes (e.g., carpeting, fabric, and wallpaper). Equally important, it may be reinforced by highlighting ordinary activities of daily living, such as food preparation in a kitchenette or small group activity around the dining room table (fig. 5.8).

Visible Activities

Activity areas are ideally located adjacent to but not a part of circulation paths (fig. 5.9) (Howell 1980). This makes activities highly visible to encourage use but does not force participation or lead to disruption. This tangential relationship also meets many of the requirements of paths for meaningful wandering.

Appropriate Group Size 2.3
Clusters of Small Activity Spaces 4.1
Public to Private Realms 4.5

Related Principles

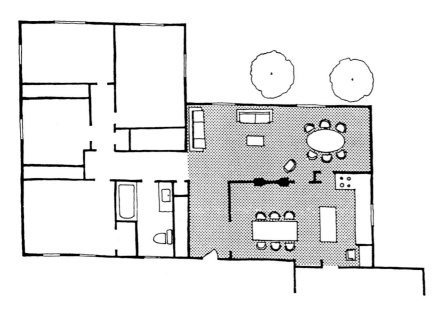

Figure 5.8
In this community-based residential facility, the common area has been subdivided to accommodate a kitchen, activity area, dining room, and family room at a domestic scale. Common activities of daily living in the kitchen further serve to enhance the residential character of the common spaces in this facility.

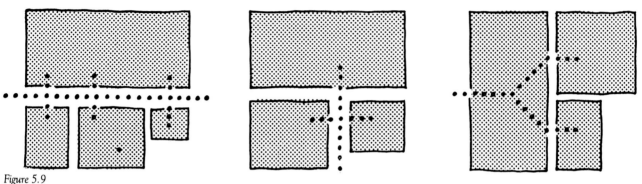

Figure 5.9
Here are three options for the arrangement of circulation paths through activity areas. The first two options allow visual access to adjacent ongoing activities without requiring participation or interruption due to intrusive circulation, as illustrated in the third diagram. (After Howell 1980.)

5.3 Domestic Kitchens

Domestic—small-scale, residential—kitchens in the home and in congregate living environments offer more than a place for essential food preparation. Accessible and safe kitchen areas for use by people with dementia make available many meaningful and therapeutic activities and experiences, including familiar household tasks, a pleasant domestic ambience, and comfortable opportunities for socialization and reminiscence.

Needs and Goals

People with Dementia

- *Need to continue familiar activities.*

- *Need to maintain a sense of control over their lives and activities.*

- *Need to maintain sense of self-esteem and utility.*

Organizational Needs

- *Need for instrumental and convenient food preparation.*

- *Need for observation and supervision of people with dementia.*

People with Dementia

As much as possible, environments and activities for people with dementia should resemble those with which residents have been familiar throughout their lives. For people with dementia, especially older women, many of their most familiar activities and experiences may have taken place in the kitchen. It is important to maintain for as long as possible these activities of daily living and the sense of utility, pride, and self-esteem often associated with food preparation and domestic chores.

Organizational Needs

Caregivers in private residences and those in formal facilities share many of the same "organizational" needs. The utilitarian need for food preparation is primary. This is a practical task that must be accommodated in some fashion, and many facilities can maximize the positive benefits of providing a role for people with dementia in this activity. Although most long-term care and congregate living environments will have a central, "functional" kitchen for large group food preparation, a domestic kitchen in the household itself can respond to many diverse, additional needs.

Facility administrators and residential caregivers also share the need for convenience in accomplishing many tasks that could easily be delegated to the household kitchen (e.g., snack and beverage preparation, table setting, dish washing). Both organizational and residential caregivers must facilitate passive, unobtrusive observation and supervision of people with dementia, preferably in a natural center of activity.

Therapeutic Goals

Safety and security are among the most pressing therapeutic goals, as the kitchen usually contains equipment and utensils that are potentially dangerous for the person with dementia. Monitoring of these items must be resolved if the kitchen is to be open to (or even provided for) people with dementia. However, the kitchen is also the setting for a host of possible activities and experiences that will be both familiar and therapeutically beneficial, meaningful, and challenging. These experiences can serve to instill feelings of autonomy, independence, and pride in achievement. These benefits surely outweigh the effort involved in making the kitchen usable and safe for people with dementia.

Organizational Goals

Administrators must ensure that organizational policies and design facilitate and enhance convenience in the care of people with dementia. To this end, a small kitchen on the unit may be appropriate if it can be used for snack and beverage preparation, thereby saving time spent traveling to a larger, generalized dining area or transporting food to individual households. A noninstitutional image benefits the facility by making the environment more attractive to residents, caregivers, and family members, all of whom are likely to respond positively to a domestic or noninstitutional ambience. Organizations have a responsibility to ensure adequate supervision of all residents and to provide opportunities for surveillance that are unobtrusive to residents without being overly demanding of caregivers. The domestic kitchen can assume the role of the conventional nurses' station.

The Kitchen as an Activity Area

A kitchen or kitchenette can easily become a major center of activity in the home or facility. In the home, the kitchen is essential for food preparation; this will not be the case in the facility, where the household kitchenette is not intended to replace the large, central, institutional kitchen. However, the kitchenette can be used as a place where residents prepare their own beverages and snacks, do dishes, sweep, and engage in other familiar domestic tasks (fig. 5.10).

Many tasks that ordinarily take place in the kitchen, such as washing vegetables, setting tables, folding dish towels, baking and decorating cookies, or making ice cream, can become the focus of group activity. A great variety of complicated and/or time-saving appliances (e.g., automatic dishwasher, food processor) are neither necessary nor advisable. Many time-consuming tasks (e.g., chopping food, hand-mixing batter, washing plates) can be quite therapeutic, as they require concentration and fine-motor skills.

From Smart Stoves to Shallow Shelves

One of the major concerns in opening the kitchen to people with dementia is the issue of safety. There are certainly many appliances and utensils that could

Therapeutic Goals

- *Ensure safety and security.*
- *Provide associations with the healthy and familiar.*
- *Support functional ability through meaningful activity.*
- *Provide regulated stimulation and appropriate challenge.*
- *Encourage autonomy and control.*

Organizational Goals

- *Reduce the institutional image of the facility.*
- *Ensure adequate supervision of residents.*
- *Strive for convenience.*

Design Concepts

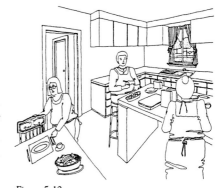

Figure 5.10
The continuous kitchen counter, the kitchen island, and proximity to the dining table allow many residents to participate in a variety of simple activities, guided and assisted as necessary by a staff member.

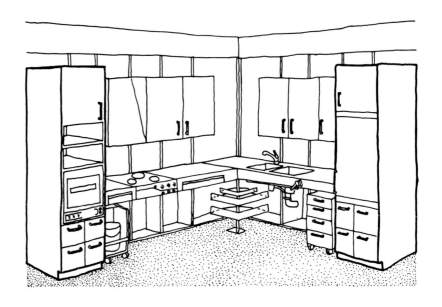

Figure 5.11
A fokus society (Sweden) adaptable kitchen. This kitchen is designed for the less able person but could also be adapted to the needs of persons with dementia. For example, it can accommodate accessible but controlled, lockable cabinets side-by-side with open shelving with viewable contents.

Figure 5.12
Simple adjustments in shelf height and depth are an example of a direct response to the changing abilities and needs of persons with dementia and their caregivers (after Goldsmith 1976).

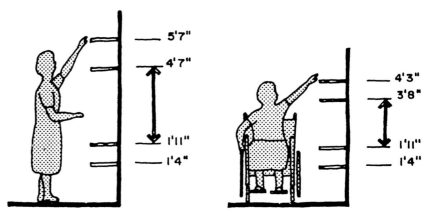

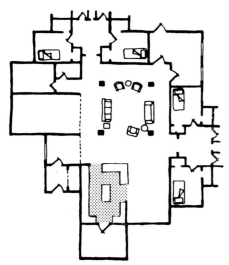

Figure 5.13
The location of the kitchen and its primary work areas allow a stationary caregiver to scan visually most of the public areas in this group home.

be misused, and some caregivers may feel that it is easier simply to lock the kitchen or not to provide one in a facility than to undertake modifications to make the kitchen safe and accessible. However, many of the potential modifications in the kitchen are relatively simple and inexpensive (fig. 5.11), and the important and meaningful experiences that can be provided in this familiar, domestic environment (especially for people in the early stages of the disease) make such changes important and worthwhile.

Instead of restricting access to the kitchen in the absence of a caregiver, it may be possible to store dangerous utensils and equipment in a single locked cupboard, leaving the rest of the kitchen open for people to get a cup of coffee or glass of water at any time, thereby providing autonomy and control. Smart stoves that turn themselves off or that require the use of an additional, inaccessible switch for operation are another attractive option. To avoid accidents, shelving units over or under work surfaces should be minimized in favor of shallow shelving units at an accessible height (fig. 5.12). Floor surfaces should be nonslippery and lighting levels high.

Unobtrusive Vantage Point

A sensitively designed kitchen work island or table can serve as an excellent center for unobtrusive observation of the household or public areas of the home. Here, the caregiver can sit or stand and supervise activities, at the same time keeping an eye on residents in the adjacent area or moving through living and dining rooms (in an open-plan home) (fig. 5.13). A telephone can be located nearby, and typical nursing-station items (paperwork, medications) can easily be stored in lockable cabinets, out of reach of residents.

The Kitchen as a Social Center

Most people are familiar with the notion of the kitchen as the "hearth" or hub of activity in the family. This can also be true for the kitchen in a facility for people with dementia. Sufficient tables should be provided to allow seating for the majority of the members of the household, preferably at familiar kitchen tables or work islands. Because the kitchen is a convenient observation post for the caregiver, it also provides a natural opportunity for informal socialization between caregivers and residents. Both residents and caregivers will enjoy the chance for coffee breaks, snacks, and conversations in this homey and comfortable place, which should be designed to enhance this image (fig. 5.14).

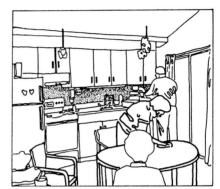

Figure 5.14
A small kitchenette and an adjoining dining room serve sixteen residents in a long-term care facility. The kitchenette does not replace the full-service kitchen; however, beverage-making, snack preparation, and the like add to the domestic character and serve as catalysts for social activities.

Noninstitutional Character 3.1
Eliminating Environmental Barriers 3.2
Intimate Dining 5.4

Related Principles

Goldsmith, S. (1976). *Designing for the Disabled.* London: RIBA Publications Limited.
Calkins, M. (1988). *Design for Dementia.* Maryland: National Health Publishing.

Additional Reading

Smaller or satellite dining areas can contribute to a greater sense of intimacy and create an ambience that is domestic rather than institutional. Such residential character can be created by ensuring a small scale and size for dining areas through the use of artifacts, varied sensory cues, and greater flexibility in scheduling and serving of meals.

5.4 Intimate Dining

People with Dementia

Snyder (1984) observed that loss of ability to feed oneself can be traumatic and can seriously decrease feelings of self-worth. Increased difficulty in the manipulation of utensils leads to frustration and negatively affects the desire and capacity to feed oneself (Hiatt 1981; Roach 1984). This, along with the overstimulation that may result from too many people and too much noise, can make mealtimes extremely stressful to and demanding of the individual, requiring great degrees of concentration and possibly leading to agitation and

Needs and Goals

People with Dementia

- *Dining has the potential for considerable trauma and stress.*

- *Overstimulation can result in agitation.*

confusion. Considering these several factors, Laxton (1985) suggested that small eating areas can minimize confusion.

Therapeutic Goals

- *Maintain ties with the healthy and familiar.*
- *Regulate sensory stimulation and provide appropriate challenges.*
- *Provide opportunities for individuality, privacy, and control.*

Therapeutic Goals

Mealtime is a potentially social, as well as nutritional, activity. Maintenance of eating patterns developed over an individual's lifetime can provide continuity with the past and increase the scope for reminiscence, an important component in the lives of people with dementia.

Small dining areas may allow more opportunities for flexible scheduling, autonomy, and control over stimulation if residents with various needs are assigned to environments with differing levels of stimulation. For example, residents could eat at their choice of three scheduled dining times in the household dining room. Family style dining could be used to allow the most competent residents to serve themselves, and staff members could serve less competent residents. When feasible, people with dementia might exercise some choice in meals by selecting between options or by providing suggestions for meals.

Design Concepts

Smaller Size

Dividing the dining room into separate subrooms or zones can reduce the institutional character associated with large dining rooms seating great numbers of people at large tables. Territorial markers, such as low partitions and plants, can define these zones, ensuring privacy for diners. Smaller groups of tables can support wayfinding behavior by breaking up a larger activity area and making the dining room portion of the space recognizable (fig. 5.15).

Small tables seating family-sized groups of two to six people can evoke associations of home, be comfortable to residents, and be more manageable for staff. Maintaining visual contact with other diners at large tables can strain neck and back muscles. Smaller tables are therefore more comfortable to residents and promote better social interaction.

Domestic Ambience

Noninstitutional furniture, such as small, square wooden tables, together with a residential decor, such as drapes and furnishings donated by residents, can serve to personalize dining areas and create a more domestic ambience (fig. 5.16). Touch and smell, as well as vision, can be used to reinforce this domestic atmosphere. Noninstitutional materials, textures, and finishes (e.g., woven placemats, carpeting on the floors) will create a residential look and feel. Cooking aromas can deinstitutionalize the dining area (and the path that leads to it) by circulating enticing smells to lead residents to the dining area and to stimulate their appetites.

Enticing Eating

In general, people with dementia tend to lose weight as the disease progresses, making dining and continuation of regular eating patterns extremely impor-

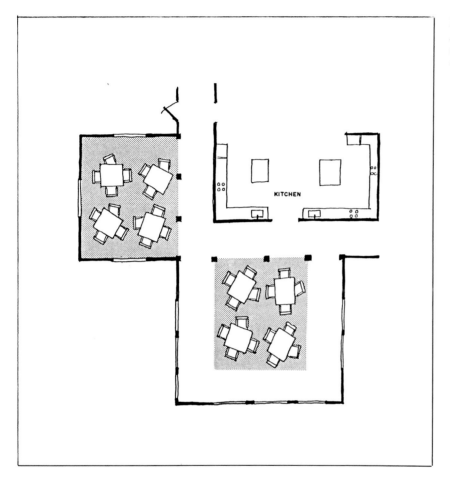

Figure 5.15
A large dining room in a long-term care facility demonstrates the concept of clear zoning and well-defined small dining areas.

KITCHEN

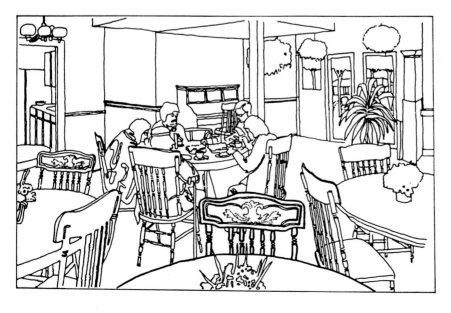

Figure 5.16
The wooden tables and chairs, plants, lighting, and small scale of the dining room create a residential and homelike environment. (Captain Clarence Eldridge Home, Hyannis, Mass.; Barry Korobkin and Associates, Architects.)

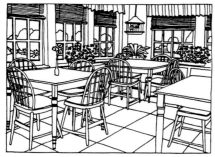

Figure 5.17
The simple organization of this small dining room, coupled with the ability to limit external stimuli by simply pulling down the shades, allows controlled stimulation at mealtime. (Wesley Hall, Chelsea, Mich.)

tant. However, dining can often be a confusing and frustrating experience for people with dementia, in part because of the large number of other people in the area and the number of distractions, including piped music or television, other residents, and windows to the outside or views of other activities that present an attractive diversion from eating. Dining is therefore one activity for which a "focused environment" may be useful; regulating stimulation in this environment may allow people with dementia to concentrate and keep them attentive to finishing their meal.

Dining areas should therefore be designed to focus on the eating experience. Possible suggestions include hanging pictures of food on the walls to remind people that it is mealtime, reducing the number of possible distractions by turning off music or television, reducing the number of other people with whom the person with dementia must have direct contact, pulling drapes temporarily to minimize distracting views to the outside, and using those types of utensils that can help people to see their food clearly (e.g., contrasting placemats and colored plates that contrast with food and table) (fig. 5.17).

Since dining areas will often also be used for other activities, it may be necessary to devise some obvious way to signal mealtime. For example, putting tablecloths on the tables in the activity area may convey that it is now mealtime; piped music and views to the outdoors, which may be pleasant during other activities, could be regulated during dining if these seem distracting to people with dementia. It is important to remember that sources of distraction will vary among individuals.

Related Principles	Eliminating Environmental Barriers 3.2
	Domestic Kitchens 5.3

5.5 Activity Alcoves

Activity alcoves can serve multiple functions by reinforcing small-group activities, providing opportunities for intimacy and retreat, and encouraging at least passive participation among people with dementia. Some characteristics of good design for activity alcoves include well-defined boundaries, a sense of closure, some suggestion of the activities that are contained within the space, and a location near or overlooking adjacent activities or paths.

Needs and Goals

People with Dementia

- *Potential confusion between day and night.*

- *Decrease in desirable interpersonal distances.*

People with Dementia

It is not uncommon for people with dementia to confuse or reverse day and night, sleeping during the daytime and subsequently wandering or lying awake during the night. It is important to provide places, other than residents' bedrooms, for rest and retreat to help mitigate this potential confusion between day and night.

There is often a decrease in the desired interpersonal distance (the amount of space desired between oneself and others in social interactions) among elderly people in general. Most people with dementia fall within this population. For this reason, large undifferentiated social spaces like dayrooms may not provide the desired sense of closeness or intimacy.

Therapeutic Goals

People with dementia may vary greatly in response to sensory and social stimulation, but overstimulation can be particularly stress-inducing (Heston & White 1983). Small social spaces, like activity alcoves, can regulate some of the overstimulation inherent in large common spaces utilized by an overwhelming number of people. In addition, activity alcoves provide opportunities for social interaction with a small group of residents or visitors or for retreat and withdrawal for residents who seek a lower degree of interaction and stimulation (Snyder 1984). Such a range of spaces and the ability to choose among them can contribute to a sense of autonomy, privacy, and control for people with dementia (Coons 1985).

Therapeutic Goals

- *Regulate stimulation and provide appropriate challenge.*

- *Foster a sense of individuality, privacy, autonomy, and control.*

Physical Closure and Boundary Definition

Activity alcoves do not need to take the actual physical form of alcoves. It is more important that these spaces provide a sense of closure and clear boundary definition in whatever form they take. Boundaries may be physical, such as a railing, or may be implied, as in the use of a different carpet color to define a particular area. Some possible physical forms of activity alcoves might include a large bay window, a small room near a path that has been converted for use as a small-scale common space, or a differentiated space within a larger area (e.g., a gazebo activity alcove within a larger public space) (fig. 5.18).

Design Concepts

Activity Alcoves as Focal Points

Activity alcoves can serve as latent landmarks for wayfinding (Weisman 1987). They may acquire such landmark status by including distinctive archi-

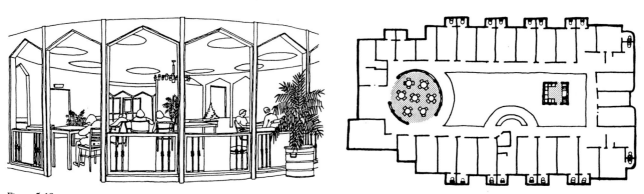

Figure 5.18
In addition to obvious "found spaces" such as bay windows, activity alcoves can be constructed in large spaces by the use of semitransparent structures such as a gazebo (a) or through the use of light railings and a canopy to define a dining room (b). (Weiss Institute, Philadelphia Geriatric Center.)

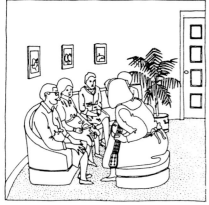

Figure 5.19
The image of the "music corner" can be reinforced by the repeated use of the place as such. The furnishings can reinforce the task and the definition of the space. The semicircular couch is used for small group music activities.

Figure 5.20
An outdoor alcove is located adjacent to a wandering path, overlooking the entire outdoor courtyard. The same idea can be used to create indoor alcoves overlooking ongoing activity areas.

tectural elements and accommodating unique activities (Coons 1985; Kromm & Kromm 1985) (fig. 5.19).

Paths That Pass By, Not Through

To allow residents to observe activities and choose appropriate levels of stimulation, activity alcoves should be created adjacent to but not part of circulation paths (fig. 5.20). Residents may then preview activities without actually entering a space and committing themselves to a social situation (Howell 1980).

Views to the Outside

While activity alcoves should be small to project domestic imagery and character and somewhat secluded to allow privacy, they should not be confining or completely enclosed, as this may be unsettling to people with dementia (Laxton 1985). Views to the outside can create a feeling of openness and provide a form of passive visual stimulation within a small space (fig. 5.21). Retreat type alcoves should be oriented toward the outside, rather than toward indoor, activity-centered areas.

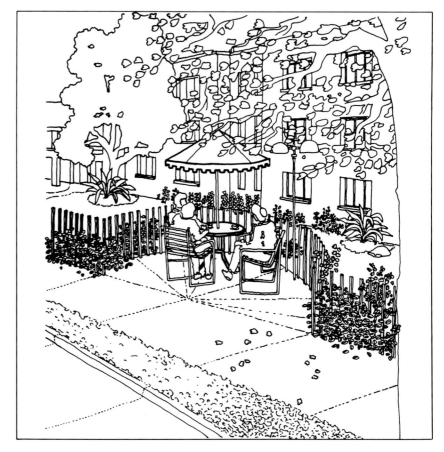

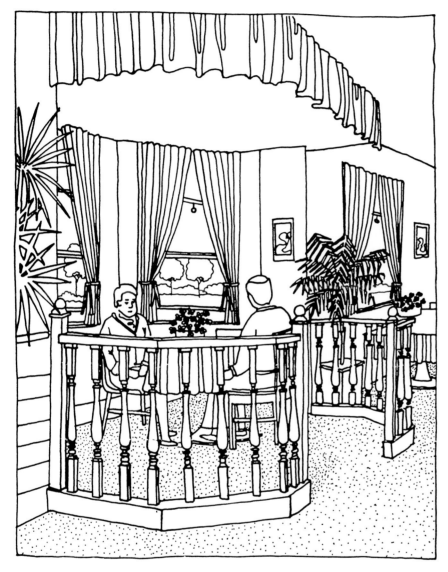

Figure 5.21
The windows in this alcove reinforce the defini-
tion of a "room," bring in natural light, and
provide a strong orientation to the outside.

Sensory Stimulation without Stress 3.4
Public to Private Realms 4.5

Related Principles

5.6 Resident Rooms

In single family homes, bedrooms are typically considered part of the most private region of the house, the area where the activities of sleeping, grooming, dressing, and personal hygiene occur. Other personal and semiprivate activities (e.g., conversation with family members, sewing, and crafts) take place in separate semiprivate spaces such as family rooms and dens. However, in many residential facilities for people with dementia, the absence of a continuum of public to private spaces means that resident rooms must accommodate both private and semiprivate activities. Conflicts between these two distinct categories of behavior can be avoided by providing separate spaces for each or significantly redesigning the typical resident room to accommodate both private and semiprivate functions.

Needs and Goals

People with Dementia

- *Relocation may disrupt continuity with one's past life.*

People with Dementia

The transition from one's own home to a group living situation can be extremely stressful. People with dementia are often removed from their everyday social support network of family and friends, as well as from the familiarity of home, neighborhood, and, in some cases, community. In these circumstances, it is essential for resident rooms to maintain continuity with those social, organizational, and physical aspects of the environment that represent a lifetime of experience for people with dementia.

Organizational Needs

Facilities for people with dementia must function within economic and regulatory constraints. These constraints often translate directly into a decision to provide shared resident rooms accommodating a broad range of activities, including treatment. However, other approaches to planning and design may also meet residents' needs for privacy as well as organizational demands for flexibility and economy.

Therapeutic Goals

- *Provide opportunities for privacy.*

- *Provide opportunities for autonomy and control.*

- *Reinforce ties with the healthy and familiar.*

- *Provide opportunities for socialization.*

Therapeutic Goals

Sleeping, grooming, dressing, and bathing are among the most private activities in the life of an individual. The need for and right to privacy should be recognized in both physical design and organizational policy. Similarly, people with dementia should retain maximal feasible control over these most private spaces. This can include choice of and control over materials, wall finishes, and furnishings, as well as use of space. Consistent with the principle of providing a continuum of public to private realms, the elimination of conflict between spaces for private and semiprivate activities can help prevent psychological withdrawal, which inhibits meaningful social interaction. The provision of privacy, autonomy, and control, and the fostering of social interaction, serve to maintain the ties of people with dementia to that which is healthy and familiar.

Design Concepts

A Place of One's Own

Rooms in residential facilities may serve as home for people with dementia for a number of years. It is essential that both physical design and organizational policy respond to the needs of such extended occupancy. Provision of semiprivate spaces has been viewed as essential to the residential qualities of long-term care facilities (Koncelik 1979). These semiprivate spaces can be incorpo-

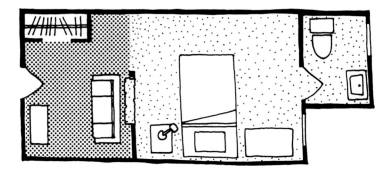

Figure 5.22
A private resident room can benefit from a continuum of zones for semiprivate and private activities. In this example, sleeping, toileting, and grooming, the most private activities, are located at the most remote and private zone within the room, whereas a space for socialization with family and friends occupies the semiprivate region near the entry.

rated either within the room or as a buffer between private resident rooms and the public corridor. Conceptually, the notion of the intimacy gradient and a continuum from public to private can be applied to the resident room as well as to the facility as a whole. Thus, the private activities of sleeping, toileting, and grooming can be accommodated in the most secure and private zone within a room, whereas spaces for reading and social interaction with family and friends might occupy semiprivate regions near the entrance to a resident's room (fig. 5.22). A second option simply moves the semiprivate space out of the residents' room and creates a separate porchlike space to serve as a transition between public and private realms (fig. 5.23). Provision of such an in-between space protects the privacy of resident rooms and can also encourage passive participation by residents in ongoing activities (Lawton, Leibowitz & Charon 1970).

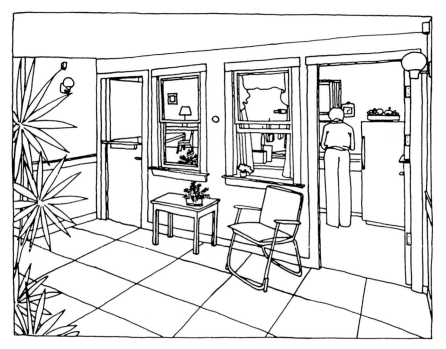

Figure 5.23
A porch-like transition zone in front of resident rooms creates a semiprivate area for socialization, as well as the opportunity for passive involvement in ongoing activities. (Captain Clarence Eldridge Home, Hyannis, Mass.; Barry Korobkin and Associates, Architects.)

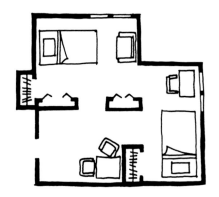
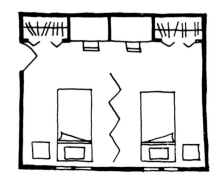

Figure 5.24
Two-resident shared rooms can be designed to create defined territories for each in response to privacy needs, at the same time retaining a semiprivate space for social contact.

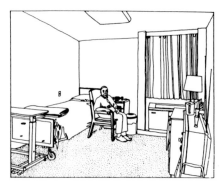

Figure 5.25
Typical institutional resident room with a lack of homelike elements or any items that can contribute to a sense of ownership.

Roommates

Residents in facilities for people with dementia typically share a room with one or more other residents; private rooms are quite scarce. Some caregivers argue that private rooms increase isolation and hasten decline; others maintain that all individuals have a need for privacy and that social stimulation can best be provided in places other than a resident's room (Ohta & Ohta 1988). While there are no hard data, practitioners seem to favor provision of private rooms to the extent possible. A number of shared rooms should be provided for individuals who prefer them (fig. 5.24), and the matching of roommates should take into consideration the personality and temperament of each.

Creating Personalized Spaces

Introduction of personal belongings and domestic furnishings can contribute to reminiscence and links with one's past and also provide useful cues for recognizing one's own room. Some measure of resident responsibility for furnishing and arrangement of the room can contribute to a sense of ownership and control (figs. 5.25 and 5.26). For example, residents might be encouraged to select their own curtains and bedcoverings and to bring a favorite chair, lamp, or dresser from home. Favorite photographs or pictures on the wall can also make the room more familiar and cheerful.

Personal Storage

Where two residents share a room, it is important that each have separate storage space (closets, drawers) for clothing and other personal possessions. Clear identification of individual possessions may minimize problems of residents rummaging through others' possessions (fig. 5.27). Conversely, built-in storage is less readily identifiable and may aggravate problems of recognition and increase institutional character.

Related Principles
Public to Private Realms 4.5

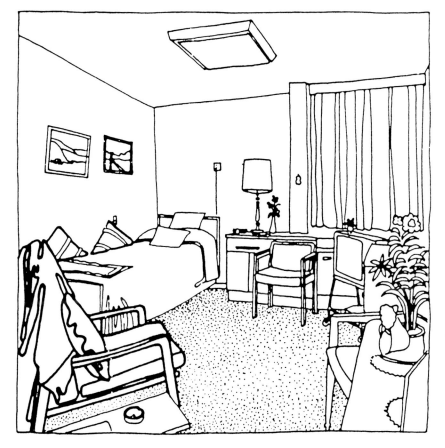

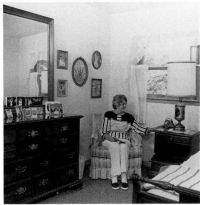

Figure 5.26
A private resident room that provides opportunities for personalization by the resident may help to foster a more familiar and homelike environment. The television set, bed pillows, and afghan are favorite familiar possessions of this resident.

Figure 5.27
Use of distinctive dressers and chests can help residents identify their possessions and also provide meaningful links to the past.

5.7 Dignified Bathing

Bathing is typically considered a difficult and trying activity for people with dementia and their caregivers. However, with sensitive design and policy decisions, it can also be viewed as an opportunity to exercise independence and preserve a sense of dignity. Places and furnishings for bathing should allow people with dementia to assume responsibility for a greater part of their own personal care, when this is possible, and to retain a sense of autonomy and of privacy under most circumstances. Accessible and sensitively designed places and equipment should also ensure that the activity of bathing be safe for people with dementia and efficient for caregivers, when they are involved.

People with Dementia

Bathing is often one of the most difficult activities performed by people with dementia and their caregivers. Because of physical deficits (including psychomotor deficits that may affect the sense of balance) and decreased attention to personal grooming, the person with dementia often requires assistance in bathing or at least in getting into and out of the bathtub or shower. However,

Needs and Goals

People with Dementia

- *Decreased attention and less ability to perform personal grooming.*

- *Possible aversion to bathing.*

being lifted into a tub or shower can easily be an unsettling or even terrifying experience. In addition, residents may resent the indignity of being assisted in bathing. Many of the various institutional bathing devices (e.g., "cranes" or hydraulic lifts to hoist the resident into the tub) compound this indignity. These circumstances often combine to create a dislike of or an aversion to bathing among persons with dementia.

Therapeutic Goals

- *Ensure safety and security.*

- *Encourage functional independence.*

- *Retain ties to the healthy and familiar.*

Therapeutic Goals

There are many concerns surrounding safety and security in bathing. For example, caregivers may experience difficulty in lifting and maneuvering the person with dementia; this is especially problematic in domestic settings, where the caregiver is likely to be an elderly spouse. Fear of falling during bathing or showering may increase the avoidance of bathing among people with dementia.

Whenever possible, people with dementia should be encouraged to take responsibility for those grooming activities (including bathing, if possible) that they can still accomplish with minimal stress or anxiety. Autonomy should be facilitated; for example, a resident may need assistance to use the bathtub but could possibly take a shower independently, seated on a wooden chair in a shower with no lip and a downward sloping floor. In such a situation, independent showering may be a more attractive alternative to the resident, and this opportunity should be provided.

Much of the equipment and many of the furnishings that have been developed to make bathing easier for the caregiver (e.g., hydraulic lifts and raised bathtubs) will probably seem strange to the person with dementia (indeed, to most people). "Bathing areas should be set up to be as reassuringly familiar and smoothly operational as possible. Bathing equipment that requires [people with dementia] to be suspended in unfamiliar contraptions" will likely be perceived as strange, threatening, and undignified (Hyde 1989, 39). In addition, noisy and crowded group bathing areas do not provide a calm setting or promote dignity for residents.

Organizational Goals

- *Safety and security in bathing areas.*

- *Efficient bathing.*

Organizational Goals

Caregivers in facilities for people with dementia are concerned with minimizing the likelihood of falling in the bathing area. Another potential problem is that unsupervised wandering into bathing areas may result in accidents. Design of bathing areas must respond to these valid concerns.

Design Concepts

Negotiable and Safe Bathrooms

Accessibility and safety are major issues that must be resolved in the design and furnishing of bathing facilities for people with dementia. People with dementia may have a great fear of falling in the bathroom; however, a variety of measures can be incorporated to reduce the risk of falling, including the use of nonslippery surfaces for floors (rubber backing can keep rugs from slipping); the installation of grab bars above the tub and along the walls; the placement of a nonslip chair in the shower; the use of a textured, nonslippery surface in bathtubs and shower stalls; and the use of a floor drain and positive drainage angles to ensure that water will not collect on the floor.

Many modifications can also make bathing facilities more accessible to people with dementia and to caregivers when they are involved. These modifications do not need to be elaborate or expensive contraptions—they can be as simple as a shower stall designed without a lip or edge and with a slightly sloping floor to allow water to drain. If the doorway of the shower is large enough to accommodate a wheelchair, a person can be pushed directly into the shower and showered in the chair.

To ensure a safe bathing area, locks can be removed from doors to prevent people with dementia from inadvertently locking themselves into the bathroom while allowing them the privacy of using the bathroom alone (when feasible). In institutions, the bathing area should be designed and located so that it is not visible to solitary wanderers and cannot be entered without a staff member's awareness.

These practical modifications can be incorporated into most homes to make the bathing area safe and accessible for people with dementia (Gnaedinger 1989):

- Slip-proof the bottom of the tub or use a rubber mat.

- Install a grab bar by the tub, or clamp a grip handle to the side of the tub.

- Purchase a plasticized seat and shower hose for bathing a seated person.

- Stick some contrasting colored tape around the edge of the tub to help define its edges and depth.

- Install washable, rubber-backed bathroom carpeting to reduce the chance of slipping on a wet bathroom floor.

- Install nonskid flooring and tiles that contrast with the tub.

- Use contrasting colors in the bathroom so that the fixtures will stand out.

- Purchase a deep soap dish so that the soap will not fall into the tub or on the floor.

- Reinforce towel bars if they are used for balancing (a grab bar is better).

Space for the Caregiver

Because bathing and showering frequently require at least some degree of caregiver assistance, areas for bathing should be designed for maximal efficiency for caregivers. Efficiency can be provided without sacrificing the dignity or privacy of people with dementia. One of the ways this can be achieved is through modification of the floor plan and layout of bathing areas. For example, bathtubs can be situated so that at least two and preferably three sides are accessible to the caregiver, with enough room on the sides of the tub to allow a wheelchair to be maneuvered directly to the side of the tub (fig. 5.28). Showers should also be large enough to allow room for a caregiver to assist with showering; if the shower can accommodate a wheelchair, less physical exertion is required on the part of the caregiver because people can be show-

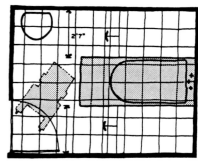

Figure 5.28
Floor plan of a bathroom with clearances that allow free movement of users and caregivers (After Goldsmith 1976).

"What I do to get her out of the tub is, first of all, I wipe up all the water from the floor with plenty of towels so it isn't too slippery; then I get her out of the tub in stages—let me tell you, that isn't easy with a wet body that doesn't cooperate—and then I prop my body, sort of wedge it between the counter and the tub, so that we won't slip and take a tumble, and then I pull her up leaning against me. There isn't room to do it

any other way. Mind you, we did have a fall one time, and got pretty bruised too!" (Husband-caregiver, age 75) (Gnaedinger 1989)

ered right in their chairs and may even be able to shower themselves without assistance. These modifications will also make the bathing area easier to clean and maintain.

Domestic and Private Bathing

To alleviate the anxieties of people with dementia, bathing should be maintained as a normal and domestic activity. When it is not possible to use familiar furnishings like residential tubs and showers, bathtubs with a "walk-in" back (fig. 5.29) are preferable to those that require the person to be hoisted over the edge. Because bathing is a private activity, group bathing areas should be discouraged, and the privacy of people with dementia should be maintained by providing shower curtains, doors, etc. For the same reason, people with dementia should be allowed to bathe themselves when possible, with the minimal assistance necessary.

Place for Grooming

Bathing and showering are activities that may require the presence or assistance of a caregiver; the same is not true, however, for grooming activities such as hair brushing, teeth brushing, make-up application, etc. Although the bathing area should be located so that it is inaccessible to solitary wanderers, the grooming area can serve as an independent activity alcove (fig. 5.30). In this way, many of the normal bathroom accessories (e.g., toothbrushes, combs) associated with grooming can be readily available to residents at all times. A special, accessible place designated for this activity may enhance residents' attention to and competence in personal grooming, reinforcing their sense of independence and self-reliance.

While regulatory standards may control the use and storage of some items

Figure 5.29
This specially designed bathtub has a removable side for entering through the gate, eliminating the need for the variety of hoisting devices used with other tubs. The bathtub also has provisions for quick filling and draining, which increase its efficiency. (Marina View Manor, HCR Inc., Milwaukee, Wis.; photographed by Tom Bamberger.)

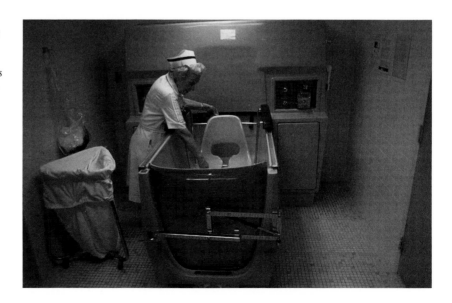

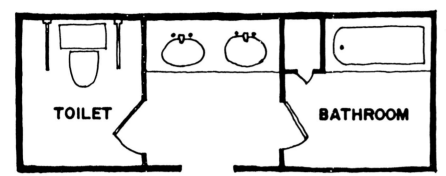

Figure 5.30
A sink and appropriate storage for toothbrushes,
etc., are part of the bathroom area but are sepa-
rate from the toilet room and the shower area.

in this area (e.g., nontoxic liquid soap instead of familiar bar soap is mandated in some states), caregivers should facilitate independence and responsibility for personal grooming activities by making hairbrushes, washcloths, etc., visible and accessible whenever possible. Clear marking and independent storage of each person's towel and toothbrush (each resident might have his or her own shelf) can lessen the confusion that often leads to "borrowing" of other residents' possessions.

Eliminating Environmental Barriers 3.2

Related Principles

Goldsmith, S. (1976). *Designing for the disabled.* London: RIBA Publications Limited.
Koncelik, J. (1976). *Designing the open nursing home.* Stroudsburg, Pa.: Dowden, Hutchinson and Ross, Inc.

Additional Reading

Although incontinence is a major problem for many people in the advanced stages of dementia, facilitating toileting can reduce this problem in the intermediate stage. Toileting areas should be designed to be easily located and identified and to be used independently by the person with dementia. These characteristics will also increase the ease with which most continent people with dementia can find and use these facilities, making toileting more dignified for all residents and making the assistance of residents a less demanding task for caregivers and staff members.

5.8 Independent Toileting

People with Dementia

Normally, toileting is considered a very private activity. However, people with dementia are often unable to locate or identify toilet facilities independently or to remember to use them without being reminded by others. Because of both the embarrassment of accidents and the need for assistance from others, toileting may become a less-than-private and dignified activity. Even upon locating the toilet area, people with dementia may have difficulty using these

Needs and Goals

People with Dementia

- *May have difficulty remembering the location of or identifying toileting facilities.*

- *May suffer from incontinence.*

115

facilities independently because of limited access or difficulty in entering and using the facilities without assistance. Incontinence becomes a major problem in the advanced stages of dementia in terms of sanitation, loss of dignity, and associated stigmatization.

Needs of Caregivers

- *Incontinence is one of the most burdensome effects of AD for the caregiver.*

- *Assisting residents with toileting can be very time-consuming.*

Needs of Caregivers

The difficulties of hygiene and housekeeping associated with incontinence are often more than the family caregiver can handle. Family caregivers report that incontinence is one of the most burdensome effects associated with Alzheimer's disease (Pynoos & Stacey 1986) and may often be a critical factor responsible for relocating people with dementia from their homes to some other setting. Incontinence is quite problematic for staff members in any type of facility for people with dementia, necessitating extra time and effort in caregiving and clean-up. In addition, assisting people with dementia in locating, identifying, and using toileting facilities is time-consuming for both professional and family caregivers.

Therapeutic Goals

- *Support functional abilities.*

- *Provide privacy and control.*

- *Assist awareness and orientation.*

- *Maintain ties to the healthy and familiar.*

Therapeutic Goals

Independent toileting is an activity of daily living that ought to be supported and extended for as long as possible. The self-esteem and dignity of the person with dementia may be closely associated with autonomy and privacy and independence in toileting. To assure independent use of toileting facilities, one must increase the visibility of these areas to people with dementia and explore alternative means of enhancing residents' awareness of the need to use such facilities. Facilities for people with dementia should also increase the relative ease of finding toileting areas, as well as employ such strategies encouraging regular toileting. Whenever possible, facilities for people with dementia should maintain the familiar appearance and usage of toileting areas, avoiding design alternatives that invade residents' privacy (e.g., group toileting areas) or that obscure the intended use of the area (e.g., a powder room or lounge area in a public restroom may obscure the function of the toileting area for some residents).

Design Concepts

Proximate and Accessible Toilet Areas

Oftentimes, problems associated with incontinence can be resolved by providing numerous toileting areas for resident use, situating these proximate to areas where residents congregate. In residential facilities, toileting areas should be associated with individuals' rooms; this will increase the likelihood that residents will be able to locate the toilet area without assistance and will use toileting facilities with relative frequency. Where it is not possible to situate a toilet and sink in each resident's room, toileting facilities should be located in immediately adjacent areas. Because toileting often follows dining, toileting areas should be located proximately but unobtrusively relative to dining facilities (fig. 5.31). In addition, restrooms placed liberally throughout a facility will reduce the time it takes for people with dementia to locate and reach a

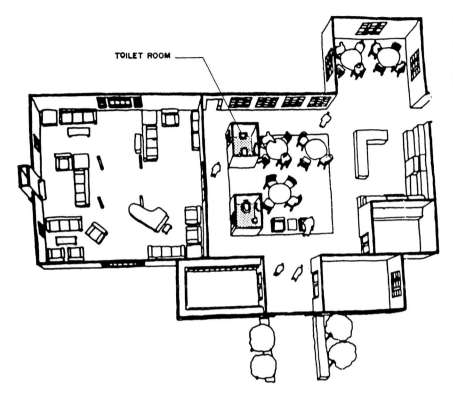

TOILET ROOM

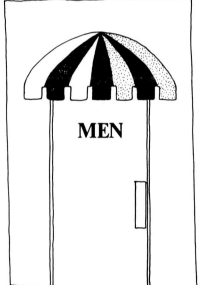

Figure 5.31
Two toilet rooms are centrally and prominently located at the core of a day care facility, near dining and activity areas. The rooms help to give definition to a wandering path, yet have unobtrusive entries.

toileting area. A large number of small restrooms located throughout the facility are more appropriate than a few large restrooms.

Recognizable Restroom

People with dementia often have trouble in locating and recognizing toileting areas. In addition to reducing the distance that residents must traverse to reach a restroom, modifications can be made that will make the restroom itself more recognizable as such. Calkins (1988) suggested the use of a line at eye level to lead residents directly from the dining area to the restroom following meals (thereby alleviating the need for residents to remember complex directions to find this area). Simple additions to the outside and door of the restroom (both the public restroom and those within the residents' rooms), when used consistently, will be recognizable cues to direct the residents to the restroom and to help them recognize it when they arrive. Such modifications might include painting the door frame and the door of the bathroom a bright, contrasting color or devising a familiar, three-dimensional marker and a large, identifiable sign to use near the door of all restrooms (fig. 5.32).

Autonomous and Private Toileting

Many modifications to toileting areas can increase the independent use of these facilities by people with dementia. For example, a simple addition—

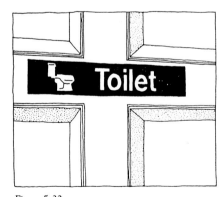

Figure 5.32
The colored canopy above the door to the restroom (a) serves as a clear marker to identify its location. The combined use of pictograms and verbal sign content (b) increases the recognizability of the room's function.

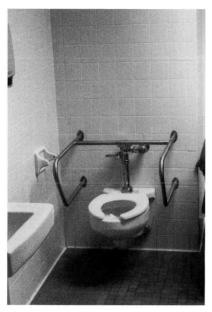

Figure 5.33
Installing grab bars next to the toilet may make it possible for the person with dementia to use the toilet independently.

such as a grab bar alongside the toilet—can alleviate the need for caregiver assistance (fig. 5.33). Private bathrooms for use by one person will be most familiar to people with dementia; where facilities for more than one person are required, independent and private toileting can still occur by providing doors (without locks) on each toilet stall to provide privacy without increasing the likelihood that people will inadvertently lock themselves into the stall. Fixtures in toileting areas should be residential and familiar to residents because people with dementia may not be able to interpret or to recognize the use of unfamiliar equipment (e.g., sink "levers," easier to manipulate than faucet handles, may be unrecognizable to residents, and so are not a wise choice in bathrooms for people with dementia).

Provisions for Wheelchair Users

In most instances, those people with dementia who are confined to wheelchairs will require some assistance in toileting. The provision of a raised toilet seat may make it easier to transfer the resident out of the wheelchair. Toileting areas that are accessible to handicapped persons should also be large enough to accommodate a caregiver and should include sufficient space for maneuvering an electric wheelchair, which requires more space than a manual chair (fig. 5.34). Because toileting is often associated with agitation and catastrophic reactions among people with dementia, finishes and surfaces that reduce reflected noise and increase sound absorbency will limit overstimulating noises that may frighten or agitate residents.

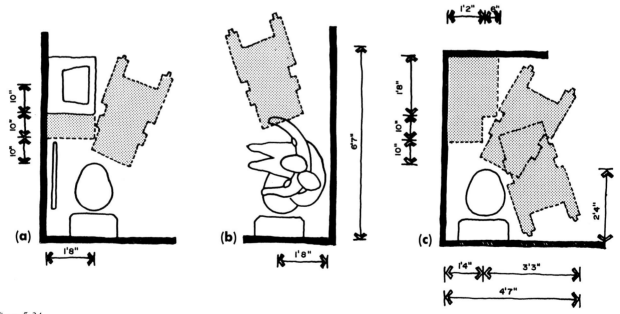

Figure 5.34
Basic space-planning requirements for toilet rooms accessible to wheelchair users: (a) relationships between water closet and sink; (b) caregiver-assisted transfer from a wheelchair; (c) wheelchair utilization space (After Goldsmith 1976).

Public to Private Realms 4.5
Dignified Bathing 5.7

Related Principles

5.9 Places for Visiting

Visits from families and friends are an important component in the lives of people residing in long-term care facilities or in group homes. It is therefore important to provide comfortable places, both public and private, for visiting. To support conversation, these spaces should be located outside resident rooms, crowded day rooms, and spaces (such as corridors) that do not readily accommodate such activities.

People with Dementia

For people with dementia in residential facilities, visiting is a critical link with the larger community. Visitors can provide people with dementia with many opportunities, such as excursions and shopping, which would otherwise be unavailable to them. Several studies also note that residents of long-term care facilities who have regular visitors tend to receive more and enhanced nursing care, presumably because visitors act on behalf of residents, often verbalizing the residents' needs when they are unable to do so (Gottesman & Bourestom 1974; Glaser & Strass 1968). Visitation also appears to have a purely therapeutic effect in itself and has been associated with decreased levels of psychological impairment among nursing home residents (Greene & Monahan 1982). Because of these benefits for people with dementia, it is important to ensure that both policy and design facilitate and encourage visiting.

Needs of Caregivers

Oftentimes, caregivers will agree to alternative residential settings (group home or long-term care facility) for the person with dementia only as a final resort, when they feel that they can no longer accommodate the person at home. Because of this, the caregiver may suffer from strong feelings of guilt; it is critical that he or she be encouraged to visit, to maintain a close relationship with the resident, and to continue to participate in the care of the family member.

Although visiting has important benefits for the person with dementia, it may sometimes be an uncomfortable experience for the visitor. Null behavior—the absence of any observable behavior or reaction—on the part of the person with dementia can leave the visitor at a loss for conversation and

Needs and Goals

People with Dementia

- *Visitors often provide important personal services.*

- *Quality of care is related to frequency of visiting.*

- *Well-being is increased by visiting.*

"Visitation is considered to have an important impact on the quality of nursing home care [and other forms of long-term care, one might presume] because it: (1) provides personal services for residents, (2) affects the amount and type of services provided by the staff, and (3) has a therapeutic influence on patient well-being." (Pynoos & Stacey 1986, 123)

Needs of Caregivers

- *Need to maintain relationship with person with dementia.*

- *Wish to feel comfortable when visiting.*

- *Need for encouragement to visit.*

things to do while visiting. In addition, the visiting family member may be dismayed to find that there is no private place available for intimate conversation or socializing. Public corridors or large, undifferentiated day rooms may appear institutional and overwhelming, and the lack of alternative, more domestic places for socializing and interaction may discourage frequent visiting. The need for such places is particularly important in those facilities where residents share a room.

Therapeutic Goals

- *Maintain links with the healthy and familiar.*
- *Promote awareness and orientation to the social environment.*

Therapeutic Goals

Continuing contact between people with dementia and their friends and family members will help to retain their ties to their past lives (fig. 5.35) and to events in the world around them. The visiting caregiver can update the resident on family news and local happenings; although the person with dementia may not remember the content of most conversations, this form of socialization can be both healthy and important for maintaining a familiar environment. This type of social interaction can also serve as a role model for other residents, who may engage in socialization more frequently when given an example to emulate (Pynoos & Stacey 1986).

Design Concepts

Range of Public and Private Spaces

Visiting can take place in many forms, from the very private and intimate (including rarely discussed but possible sexual activity) in the resident's room to some shared and public interaction between two or more families and several residents. This variety in visiting activities and circumstances calls for a range of places for visiting, responsive in terms of location, type, and related characteristics. Residential facilities for people with dementia might incorpo-

Figure 5.35
Visiting can be a happy and positive experience for people with dementia and their family members, facilitating recall of many of the experiences of home. (Jerry and Pat Schmidt; photographed by Robert Glick.)

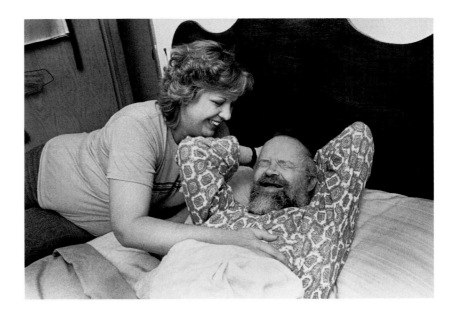

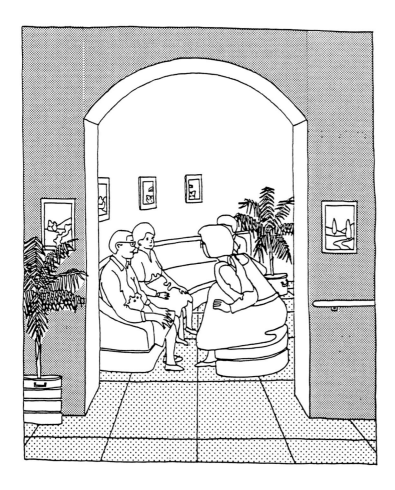

Figure 5.36
Small, semipublic spaces, such as alcoves, allow
a degree of privacy for visitors and residents.

rate some or all of the following types of spaces: private nooks or alcoves for
two or more people for intimate conversation and reflection (fig. 5.36); en-
closable dens or small rooms for visiting families and small group activities
(such as looking at photographs or playing an easy game); large, more active
public areas that offer stimulation to the person with dementia and a chance
for the visitor to participate in a nearby, ongoing activity (at this scale, even
the dining room can be a place for visiting, affording the visiting spouse or
family member a chance to participate in caregiving activities, such as helping with meals).

Friendly Domestic Image

To increase the physical and psychological comfort of visiting family members
or friends, places for visiting should be familiar and residential in scale, furnishings, and finishes. The typical "institutional" day room—easy to clean,
with high gloss floors and chairs lined up against the walls—can be replaced
with a more domestic environment, which includes carpeting, residential
chairs and sofas provided by the residents or caregivers, and cheerful decorations (fig. 5.37).

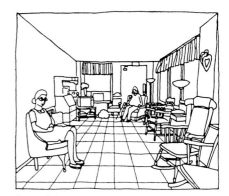

Figure 5.37
A relaxed domestic atmosphere was created in
this popular room for visiting through the use of
various recycled residential furnishings. This
domestic ambience can help both visitors and
residents to feel more comfortable.

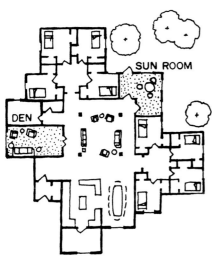

Figure 5.38
Both the sun room and the den in this eight-person group home are part of the public zone. However, the French doors that lead into both spaces can provide closure and privacy during visiting.

Multifunctional Spaces

It is not always feasible or desirable to create places that have only a single function (e.g., places for visiting or for staff retreat only). The design of multi-use spaces is clearly a useful strategy to resolve many spatial problems without compromising any necessary activities. For instance, an alcove used for music therapy can also be used for intimate gathering when therapy is not taking place. The list of potential multifunctional spaces includes activity alcoves, positive outdoor spaces, entry lobbies, sunrooms, and meeting rooms (fig. 5.38).

Things to Do

Residents in facilities for people with dementia are often extremely passive and often display null behavior. Visiting under such circumstances can become very frustrating for family members, who may find themselves simply staring at a resident with little conversation or activity actually taking place. While quiet reflection may sometimes be desirable, the provision of "things to do" during visiting can alleviate visitors' discomfort at trying to force conversation or create activity. Places for visiting can benefit from having a view to ongoing activities and action, both indoors and out. Locating these spaces adjacent to passageways to the outside would enable visitors to take a walk with a resident, thereby encouraging some level of activity. It might also be useful to provide some simple games or other activating agents, such as things from the past, that could foster conversation or reminiscence (fig. 5.39).

Related Principles	Noninstitutional Character 3.1
	Activity Alcoves 5.5

Figure 5.39
Things from the past act as catalysts for conversation with people with dementia, whose long-term memory may be relatively intact. Since conversation and socializing are the activities associated with visiting, furnishing these spaces with photo albums, familiar "old-fashioned" kitchen implements or tools, hand-made decorations, and other memorable things from the past can initiate conversation by visitors and/or residents.

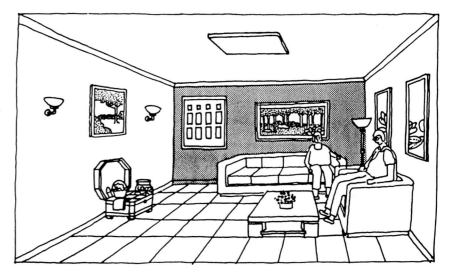

5.10 Staff Retreat

Facilities for people with dementia should include a space for staff retreat, work task completion, private conversations, socialization, and decompression. This intimate and convenient place should increase both quality of life for and feelings of community among staff members.

Staff Needs

Staff members need a place to retreat from the continuous pressure of work and contact with residents, family members, and visitors. They should be able to take a short break, pause for a cup of coffee, or relax. "Backstage" environments (Goffman 1961) for staff are places where one is not scrutinized and can let one's guard down. The lack of formality of not being "on stage" can be relaxing by itself.

In addition to this need for a place for physical and mental retreat, staff members need a place for socialization and private conversations and opportunities to meet and interact with other staff members. They also require a place where instrumental, work-related tasks that require concentration (e.g., charting) can be accomplished free from interruption.

Organizational Needs

"Frontline" caregivers for people with dementia are typically low paid, semi-skilled workers with a high turnover rate. This turnover can diminish both the efficiency of the institution and satisfaction among both remaining staff and residents. Organizations must combat employee turnover, at the same time attracting high-quality employees to their facility. Staff retreat areas can act as an important component in building a sense of worth among employees.

The provision of such spaces does not preclude staff members from enjoying their meal and break times in interaction with the residents; opportunities for both retreat and interaction should be provided, and the use of such spaces will depend upon both organizational policy and personal preference. The potential abuse of staff retreat areas as places for employees to congregate at the expense of time spent on the job must be resolved by organizational policy; however, the need for such spaces is real.

Job satisfaction for staff members can be enhanced through the provision of opportunities for temporary retreat from job pressures. Facilities for people with dementia should support the job tasks that staff members must accomplish. These may require supplementary or alternative work spaces, some of which can be incorporated into staff retreat areas. Designated places for staff retreat should enhance staff members' positive self-image. Providing opportunities for socialization with other employees at the workplace will foster team spirit and contribute to job satisfaction.

Therapeutic Goals

Staff places that are noninstitutional in nature will be familiar and recognizable to residents. This continuity between staff and resident places will help to

Staff and Organizational Goals

- *Ensure job satisfaction and quality of life.*

- *Ensure task completion.*

- *Promote a positive self and group image in employees.*

- *Provide opportunities for socialization on the job.*

- *Attract and secure the best available employees.*

Therapeutic Goals

- *Maintain ties to the healthy and familiar.*

• *Ensure the safety and security of residents.*

create a more residential environment, which can be appreciated by residents, family members, and other caregivers. Staff retreat areas can also serve as places where such potentially dangerous objects as medications and cooking or heating appliances (e.g., coffee maker, hot plate) can be stored out of the sight and reach of residents.

Design Concepts

Comfortable Lounge

The character of a staff retreat area should be such that it is both a comfortable and a comforting place to escape momentarily the pressures of the job and to relax. For this reason, staff places should provide an opportunity for privacy from residents (fig. 5.40). Places to sit and appliances for making coffee and heating food are also desirable (fig. 5.41).

Informal Image

Staff retreat areas should adopt, as much as possible, an atmosphere and character in keeping with the noninstitutional image projected for the entire facility. This design concept is targeted particularly at the elimination of the traditional nurses' control station as the primary gathering and work space for staff members (fig. 5.42). Both staff work and retreat areas should strive for an image consistent with the home environments with which employees and resi-

Figure 5.40
In this floor plan of a day care center, the staff office is separated from the activity area, yet its strategic location allows supervision of the entrance and exit from the facility.

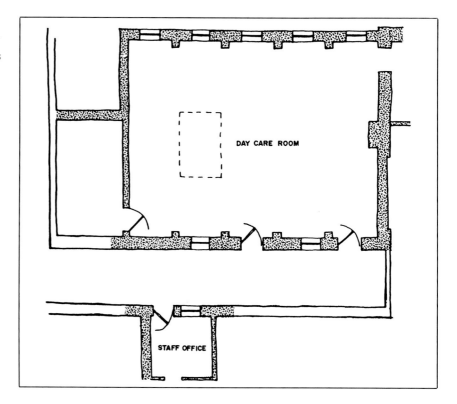

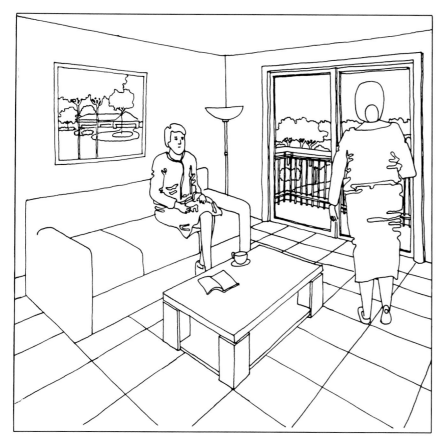

Figure 5.41
Comfortable seating, provision for snacks and coffee, and good views can make a short break a real delight.

dents are familiar. This should foster a less "medical model" organizational at-titude and a more informal relationship between staff members and residents.

Place to Work and Reflect

Staff members often need a place for private conversations and consultations and a location where they can perform work tasks that suffer from constant interruption by incoming calls, resident demands, and family members with questions or concerns. Staff members complain that truly private conversations are impossible at a busy nurses' station and that employees are perceived as rude or unresponsive when they fail to respond immediately to interruptions while charting, consulting with another staff member, etc. Staff members need a place separated from busy public areas where they can perform these necessary work tasks and activities. In keeping with the informal image advocated here, facilities might adopt a simple desk or table with a telephone and other necessities directly near the residents and move the location of other necessary work tasks and props to a separate staff work area (for tasks that demand concentration and freedom from interruptions) or a storage area (for charts, files, and medications) (fig. 5.43).

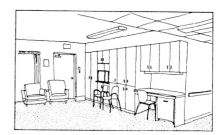

Figure 5.42
The performance of charting and other paper-work at a remote staff area reduces the conventional nurses' station in this unit to a small wall counter and a secure telephone in the corner of the living room. (The Cedar Lake Home Tri-Campus, West Bend, Wisc.)

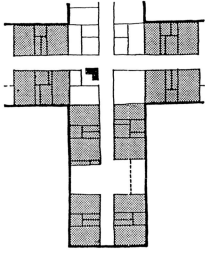

Figure 5.43
This long-term care facility developed a scheme that includes both "primary" and "secondary" nursing stations. The hub between four "households" provides a possible place for work that can be removed from the household unit. In this example, an opportunity to provide privacy is compromised by the desire to maintain visual surveillance. (The Cedar Lake Home Tri-Campus, West Bend, Wisc.)

Community Resource Center

A staff lounge area might serve as an informal center for information and resources for employees, housing such necessary resources as journals, relevant articles and announcements, notifications of changes in policy or procedure, etc. A bulletin board could be included to hold staff members' photos, cartoons, quips, and memos, and staff mailboxes would serve to draw employees. The professional and community atmosphere of the staff lounge reinforces employees' sense of community and perception of themselves as valuable members of the organization.

Multiple-Function Spaces

In most facilities, space is at a premium. Many organizations cannot afford a room that is designated for a part-time activity (such as staff retreat). A possible solution is to design a room appropriate for a number of nonconflicting functions (fig. 5.44).

Remote and Proximate Retreats

Staff retreat areas can exist in a variety of locations, both near to and away from the unit. Facility-wide dining rooms and lounges offer opportunities for socialization between employees from different units and between staff and administration, encouraging a sense of community among all employees. On the other hand, staff retreat areas located in individual units will be more easily used by unit staff members, making these areas more accessible and convenient for work tasks and continuous contact with the residents, as well as providing opportunities for team-building and socializing within the unit (fig. 5.45).

Related Principles

Noninstitutional Character 3.1
Public to Private Realms 4.5

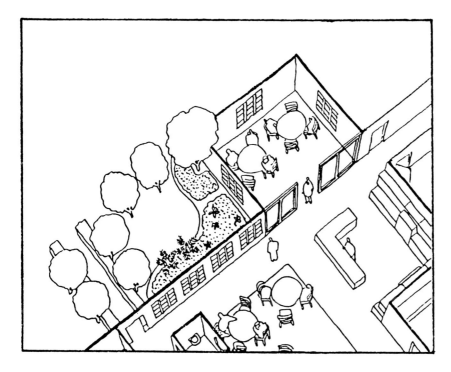

Figure 5.44
The den with French doors is adjacent to the main public area and can function as an activity alcove. With the doors closed, the den can function as a staff retreat or a place for a family visit.

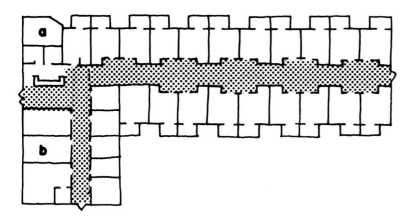

Figure 5.45
This schematic drawing of a typical nursing home shows a staff lounge on the main public area of the unit (a) and a remote lounge in the "administrative" zone (b).

Overleaf: Hanson Graphic; Martha Svendson, photographed by Tom Bamberger

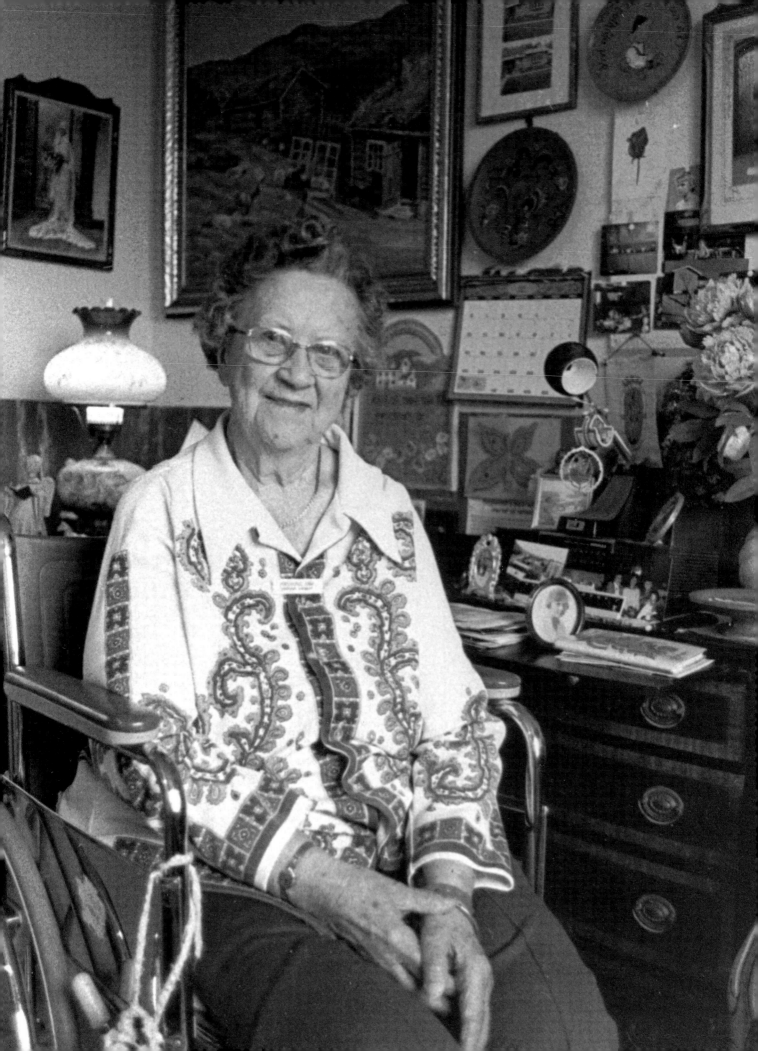

6 *Design: Prototypical Facilities*

Chapters 2 to 5 present a series of discrete principles for the planning and design of facilities for people with dementia. The effective application of such principles, however, requires their integration in the context of specific projects. In recognition of this, chapter 6 presents designs for seven prototypical facilities, ranging from a small community group home to the renovation of a nursing unit within a traditional long-term care facility.

Each facility is described in both organizational and architectural terms, beginning with a summary of structure, program, and specific design features. This is followed by an annotated overview of the complete facility, with specific building elements clearly linked to relevant principles for planning and design. In this way, relationships between basic concepts, rooted in therapeutic and organizational goals, and resultant architectural form are made manifest. The presentation of each facility concludes with a series of interior views that convey something of the desired experiential qualities judged to be appropriate to the needs of its users.

The development of these seven prototypical facilities was viewed as an opportunity to engage in inquiry by design (Zeisel 1981). This process took place in two ways: (1) by testing specific principles and assessing their value in the making of planning and design decisions and (2) by serving as a source for new and revised principles, the need for which emerged only through the planning and design process. In this spirit of inquiry by design, these seven prototypes and the principles upon which they are based should be viewed as a first rather than a final word regarding supportive environments for people with dementia. Each should be viewed as a hypothesis awaiting additional exploration and validation.

This day care center for thirty people is a freestanding building on an urban site (fig. 6.1). It is a newly constructed structure; however, the basic design elements developed for this prototype can also be applied in an addition to or a renovation of an existing facility.

6.1 Day Care Center

Organizational Requirements

- Number of clients: thirty at peak times
- Staffing ratio: one direct care staff member per four clients

Program

Figure 6.1
Day care center: bird's eye perspective.

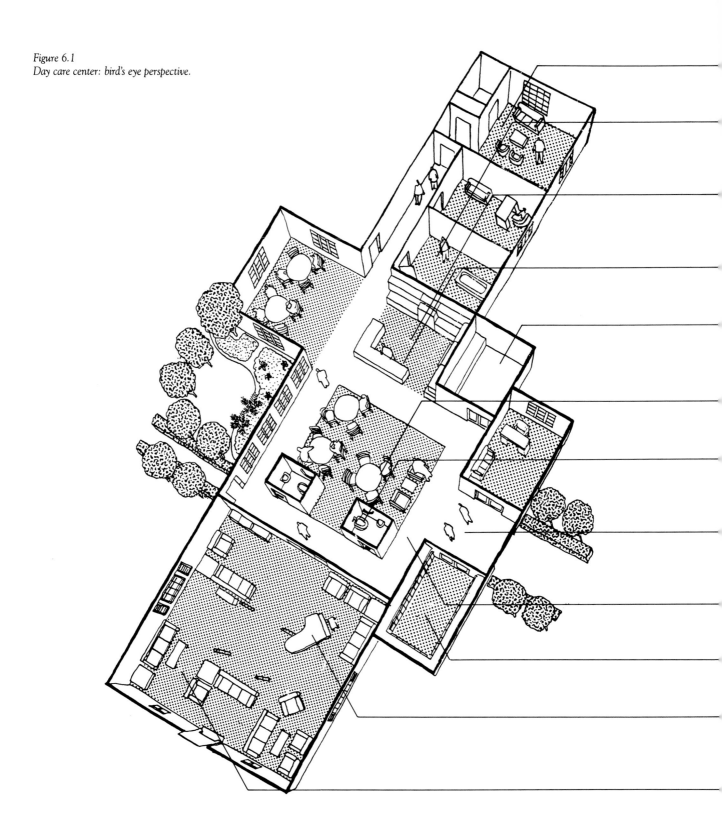

Staff retreat
Includes a lounge, separate restroom, washer and dryer, etc.

Assisted bathing area
Designed to accommodate grooming activities and bathing or showering of clients if necessary or desired by caregiver

Domestic kitchen
Designed to be used by both clients and staff as a part of the daily program of activities

Unobtrusive observation (fig. 6.2)
Clear visual access to most public spaces from kitchen island

Quiet room
Multifunctioning quiet space for retreat of agitated clients and for visiting with family members

Intimate dining areas (fig. 6.3)
Two well-defined spaces for small group dining

Legible and easily identified toilet rooms
Room enclosures with strong visual presence; easily located, yet unobtrusive from dining areas

Friendly entry
Entry sequence and cloak room that are clearly defined and provide an opportunity to preview activity areas before entering

Meaningful wandering path
Links key social spaces

Storage area/cloak room
Removed from main activity areas to discourage rummaging

Noninstitutional furnishings
Tables and chairs in small groupings to encourage contact; the piano as a valued link to the past for many clients

Activity alcoves
Living room subdivided into small, residential-scale areas

General Attributes

- Noninstitutional character
- Secure and easily accessed outdoor area
- Range of spaces from public to private
- "Friendly" entry area that allows gradual transition into the facility

Building Organization

- Visual connections between primary public areas, allowing one to see most of the facility from the entry; spaces that are not fragmented
- Separation between public areas and support or service spaces
- Wandering path surrounding core areas
- Differentiated activity alcoves within the living room

Activity Areas

- Designated locker and storage room for coats, etc.
- Dual-functioning quiet room and visiting area
- Assisted bathing area
- Domestic kitchen for client and staff use
- Unobtrusive observation of activity areas from the kitchen
- Accessible outdoor area
- Designated entry area allowing "preview" of the facility
- Administrative office space
- Staff retreat area with adjoining restroom

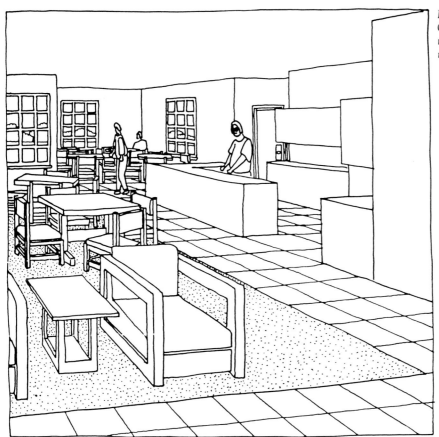

Figure 6.2
Caregivers can easily survey public areas from
the kitchen island, eliminating the need for a
traditional nursing station.

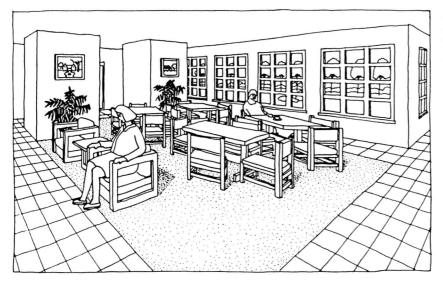

Figure 6.3
Intimate dining is encouraged through the use of
residential kitchen tables arranged in small
groups.

6.2 Day Care and Respite Center

This design solution consists of many of the basic elements introduced in the preceding design for a day care center; therefore, only those elements that are unique to the respite function are presented here (fig. 6.4). These elements include some additional activity areas (e.g., beauty shop) and those spaces that are necessary to support overnight stays.

Figure 6.4
Day care and respite center: bird's eye view.

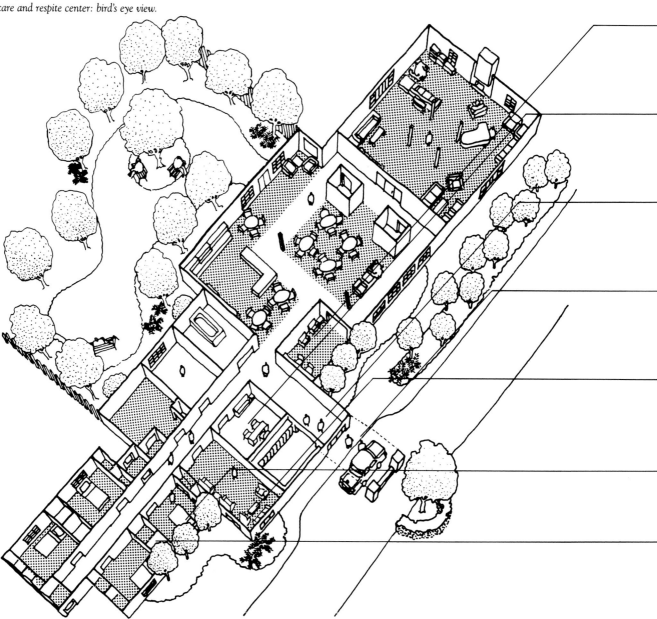

Design Responses

Beauty shop
Provides the setting for a familiar community-based activity; serves as a landmark within the center

Administrative office
Serves as reception area into facility and unobtrusive surveillance point from which to deter potential wanderers

Gradual entry and transition area
Allows moderated entry into public areas that does not interfere with ongoing activities

Sheltered and safe entrance
Provides drop-off point that is protected from the weather and does not expose clients to traffic danger

Shared space
Activity area is available to respite clients during hours when day care facility is not in operation.

Bedrooms
Four bedrooms can accommodate up to eight overnight residents at a time.

Adjoining toilet rooms
Private, familiar location of these rooms makes them easy for residents to find.

The central space (fig. 6.5) and the kitchen counter (fig. 6.6) function as in the day care center (facility 6.1).

Figure 6.5
The central space accommodates dining and informal activities and provides opportunities for wandering at the periphery.

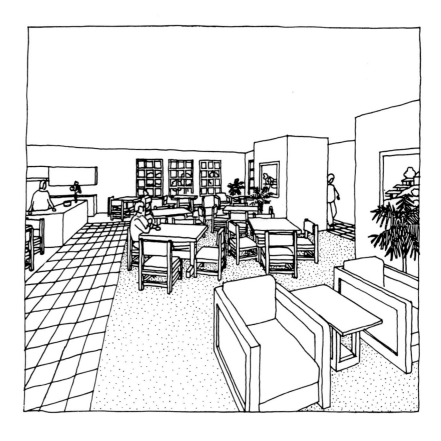

Figure 6.6
The kitchen counter provides an unobstructed view of the dining area, the entry to the living room, and an outdoor activity area.

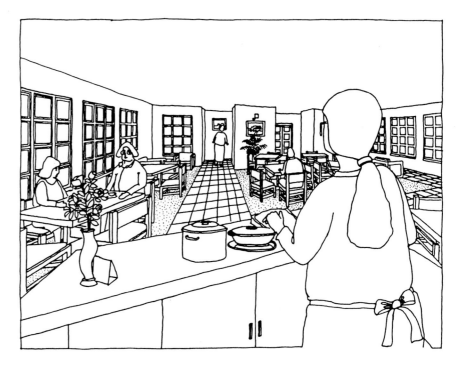

Organizational Requirements

- Number of clients: thirty at peak daytime hours, with a maximum of eight overnight residents

- Staffing ratio: one direct care staff member per four clients during daytime hours, plus one nighttime staff member

Building Organization

- Separate entrance area that does not lead directly into activity areas; persons entering and leaving do not intrude on ongoing activities.

- Entrance area provides a sheltered and secure drop-off area for clients.

Activity Areas

- Beauty shop is centrally located within day care area.

- Resident rooms with adjoining shared space can function as a self-contained unit during nighttime hours.

The group home for eight residents is a freestanding house on a suburban site (fig. 6.7). It is a newly constructed building and incorporates many design features that cannot be readily introduced into an existing house converted to a group home.

6.3 Group Home for Eight Residents

The program was developed in part by Dorothy Coons of the Institute of Gerontology at the University of Michigan, Ann Arbor.

Organizational Structure

- Number of residents: eight

General Attributes

- Noninstitutional character

- Gradation of spaces from public to private

- Links to things from the past through accommodation of familiar activities

Building Organization

- Private resident rooms with toilet and lavatory for maximal privacy

- Direct access to the outdoors

- A safe walking path extending to the outdoors, with a variety of activities and stimuli along its course

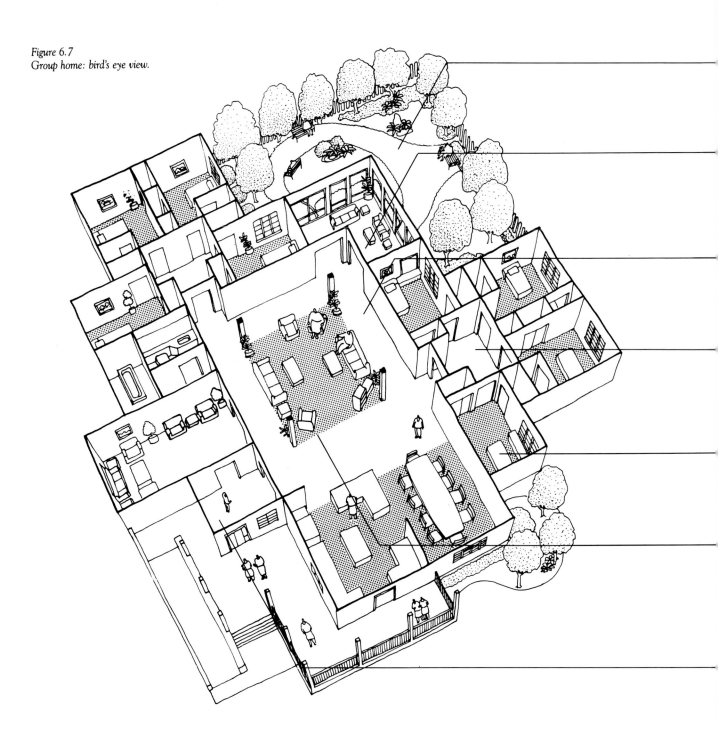

Figure 6.7
Group home: bird's eye view.

Positive outdoor spaces
Direct access to adjacent outdoor activity area

Places for visiting (fig. 6.8)
Den and sunroom can be enclosed and separated from the more public core of the facility to serve as places for visiting with family and friends.

Opportunities for meaningful wandering
Indoor walking path connecting different activity areas and key social spaces

Clustering activities and spaces
Clusters of four resident rooms around a semiprivate core, with complete elimination of corridors; public activities are clustered around a public core.

Resident rooms
Private rooms with storage and baths to ensure maximal privacy

Public to private realms
Gradation of spaces from entry to living room (fig. 6.9), dining room, and kitchen, to semipublic den and sunroom, to semiprivate zones adjacent to resident rooms to the private core of individual resident rooms

Noninstitutional character
Residential scale with resident room clusters, no corridors, elimination of the nurses' station, front porch, and exterior residential imagery

Figure 6.9
The living room can accommodate most communal activities of the home, such as holiday meals. It is the central space of the house, connected to other functions and the clusters of residents' rooms, yet it has its own spatial boundaries. Columns and bookcases define the living room and contribute to its residential character.

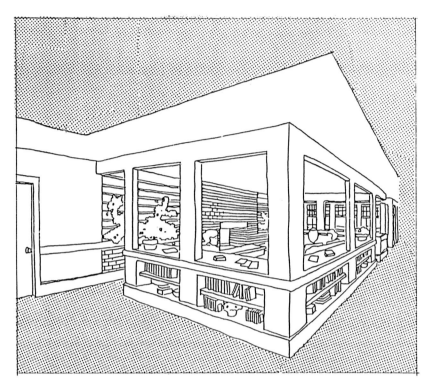

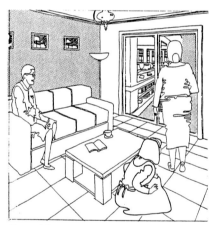

Figure 6.8
The den links the living room and its surrounding path to the outdoors. It can serve as an extension of the central activity area or, with the French doors closed, can become a private area for visiting or retreat.

- Elimination of the traditional double loaded corridor by clustering resident rooms around a common core
- Elimination of the formal "fortress-like" nurses' station

Activity Areas

- Public, shared spaces with clear identity and character, including living and activity areas, den area for quiet activities, dining area, and kitchen for both resident and staff use
- A support area including washer, dryer, heating unit, and needed storage

While accommodating more people than most group homes, this facility for twenty attempts to reduce the institutional character typically associated with facilities for a large number of residents (fig. 6.10).

6.4 Group Home for Twenty Residents

Organizational Structure

- Resident population of twenty is broken down into smaller functional groups of six or seven, with four caregivers.

General Attributes

- Noninstitutional character: facility consists of three residential-scale clusters of spaces.

Building Organization

- Opportunities for meaningful wandering through the provision of a walking path that connects various activity spaces, providing points of interest along the way
- Variety of spaces ranging from the most public areas at the facility center to semipublic shared spaces for each cluster to the private resident rooms, establishing a gradient from public to private realms
- Clustering of residents' rooms with small dining/activity areas defining functional and social groups

Activity Areas

- Shared spaces consisting of living, dining, kitchen, and pantry areas forming the core of the facility
- Clear definition of the entry sequence to the home

Program

Figure 6.10
Twenty-person group home: bird's eye view.

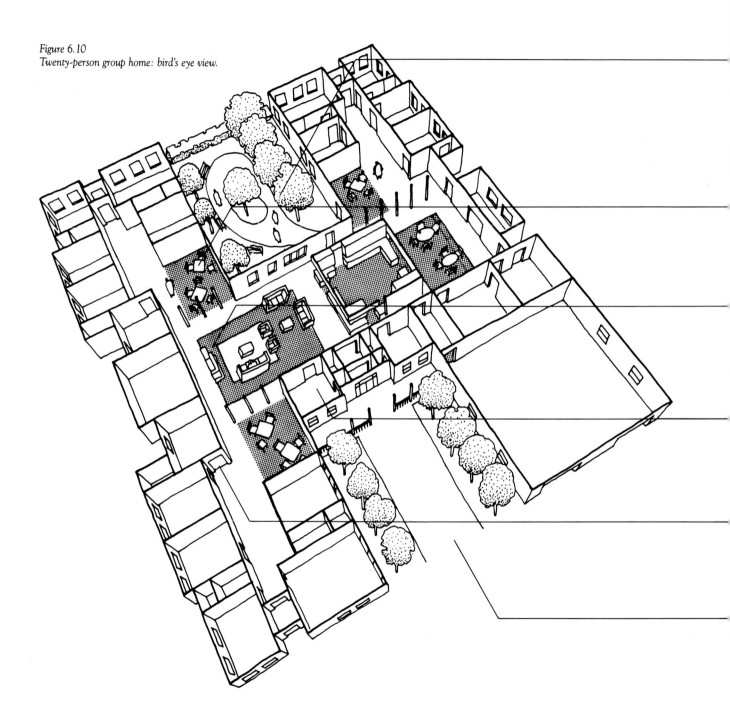

Positive outdoor space
Floor plan creates protected outdoor spaces at both the front and the rear of the home. A residential character for the entrance and a defined entry sequence are provided by the landscaping. At the rear, an outdoor space provides opportunities for meaningful activities, as well as pleasant views from resident rooms and public shared spaces into a landscaped courtyard.

Clustering activities and spaces
Rooms for seven residents and a dining/activity area (fig. 6.11) included in each cluster are residential in scale and character.

Opportunities for meaningful wandering
A wandering path connects social spaces and passes interesting activities (e.g., beauty shop, pergola) along the way, as well as providing views to the outside.

Shared spaces
The shared spaces constituting the public core include a living area, kitchen and pantry, and a beauty shop.

Public to private realms
Gradation from public shared spaces at the core of the facility to semipublic activity areas for each residential cluster to private resident rooms

Entry and transition
The entry sequence is reinforced through the front porch and vestibule, creating a transition from the outdoors to the indoors. The porch provides a semiprotected vantage point from which to observe activities on the street (fig. 6.12).

Figure 6.11
The selection and arrangement of furnishings in this group home are structured to create multi-functioning spaces for intimate dining and household-based activity areas.

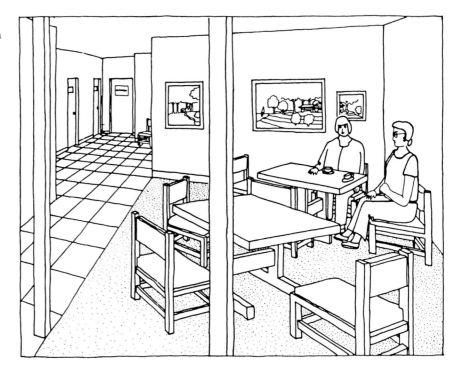

Figure 6.12
The friendly and homelike exterior signifies a familiar and comforting environment to residents and family caregivers alike.

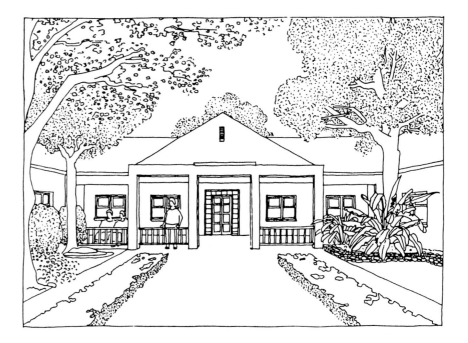

This freestanding facility can potentially function either independently or in cooperation with an adjacent nursing home. It acts as a bridge between smaller group homes and larger, more traditional long-term care facilities. This facility consists of three 12-resident households; these households can function together or can create and maintain separate identities (fig. 6.13). Thus, it would be possible to accommodate residents in three different phases of Alzheimer's disease.

6.5 Freestanding Thirty-six-Resident Facility

The program for this facility is based in part upon Woodside Place in Oakmont, Pennsylvania, a project sponsored by the Presbyterian Association on Aging and West Penn Hospital.

Program

Organizational Structure

- Resident clusters of the facility may function in either an integrative or an autonomous fashion.

- Each cluster could potentially accommodate residents at the same level of functional ability.

General Attributes

- The pinwheel floor plan, hip roofs, and courtyards all contribute to a noninstitutional character.

- The facility functions along a gradient of privacy from private to public realms (e.g., from private resident rooms to sitting and dining areas within each cluster to shared general public areas at the center of the facility).

- Single-floor organization increases overall accessibility.

Building Organization

- The L-shaped plan of each cluster defines four outdoor spaces but also results in a more traditional double-loaded corridor configuration.

- Direct access to a protected outdoor court is provided for each resident cluster.

- The living room of each cluster has potential visual access both to the outdoors and to larger, common public areas.

Activity Areas

- Each cluster has facilities for light cooking by residents, reheating prepared meals, and other possible kitchenette activities.

- The shared public zone provides opportunities for wandering.

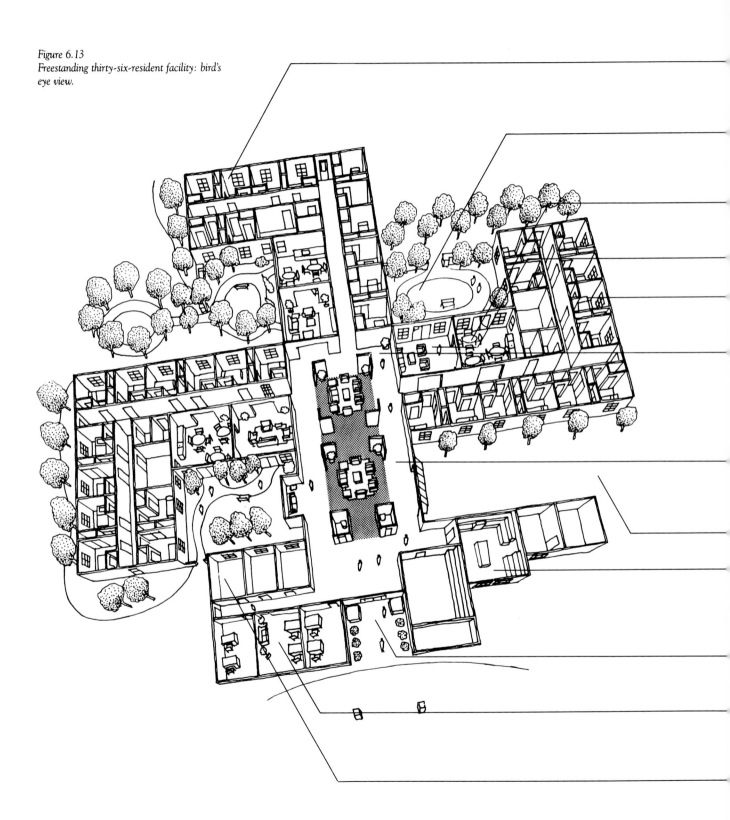

Figure 6.13
Freestanding thirty-six-resident facility: bird's
eye view.

Household clusters
These serve to structure the facility in both organizational and architectural terms.

Protected outdoor courtyard (fig. 6.14)
Each household cluster has direct visual and physical access to its own outdoor area.

Kitchenette and dining area
These are provided on an intimate scale for the residents of each cluster.

Household living room

Private bedroom with attached bathroom
Residents are able to enjoy privacy within their own rooms.

Wandering path
Connects all three clusters and surrounds common public space

Public spaces for use by all residents
Contain distinct activity areas

Activity alcoves
One of these alcoves functions as an attached greenhouse, and the other serves as a nook for visiting and watching.

Common public outdoor area

Kitchen
The size of the kitchen is dependent upon whether the facility is self-contained or associated with an adjacent long-term care home. If meals come from elsewhere, the kitchenette can function as a pantry and a place for reheating food.

Protected entrance (fig. 6.15)
Secure entrance shields residents from inclement weather.

Administrative and support spaces, as needed
These spaces serve office, storage, and laundry functions and can increase in size as needed to meet the requirements of each facility.

Guest room
For overnight use by visiting family members

Figure 6.14
Three sides of each outdoor courtyard are defined by the building itself, minimizing the need for more obtrusive types of enclosure. Living and dining spaces of each cluster have direct visual and physical access to an outdoor court.

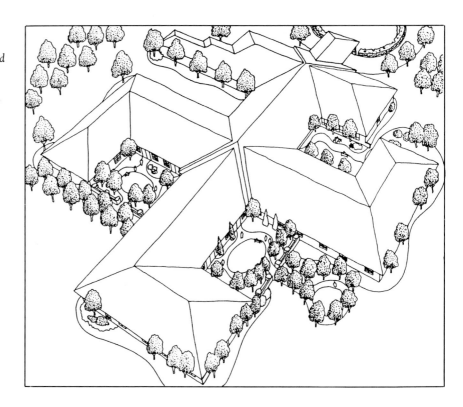

Figure 6.15
The roof of the port cochere extends over the drive, providing a sheltered and welcoming entry. Although the image of the building is not residential, it still remains noninstitutional in nature.

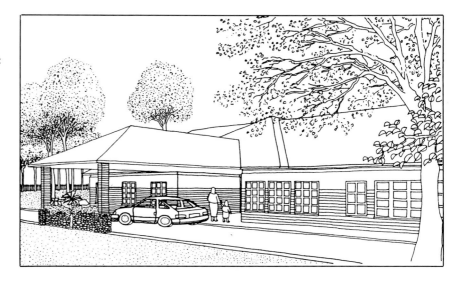

- Shared public spaces can accommodate specialized activities and events, such as music therapy, crafts, gardening in indoor raised planting beds, holiday dinners, or perhaps occasional performances by local musicians in a small auditorium.

- The administrative wing defines a large, common outdoor area for exercise and other activities that may require more space.

- Activity alcoves placed along the public wandering path can be used for visiting and solitude or can accommodate an attached greenhouse.

This design illustrates the restructuring of an existing nursing unit in a long-term care facility. The original twenty-four-bed unit is converted into a self-contained eighteen-bed nursing unit, which includes a dining area and shared social spaces (fig. 6.16).

6.6 Renovation of a Long-term Care Facility

Organizational Structure

- Number of residents: eighteen

- Self-contained special care unit accommodating all dining, social, and therapeutic activities

General Attributes

- Noninstitutional character; effort to minimize preexisting institutional character

Sensory Stimulation

- Increasing the level of sensory stimulation to engage the interest and competence of residents

Building Organization

- Small, defined spaces for shared activities form a social core and also eliminate the long corridor with identical doors lining each side.

- Secure access to the nursing unit

Activity Areas

- Opportunities are provided for outdoor activities.

- Resident rooms remain semiprivate.

Program

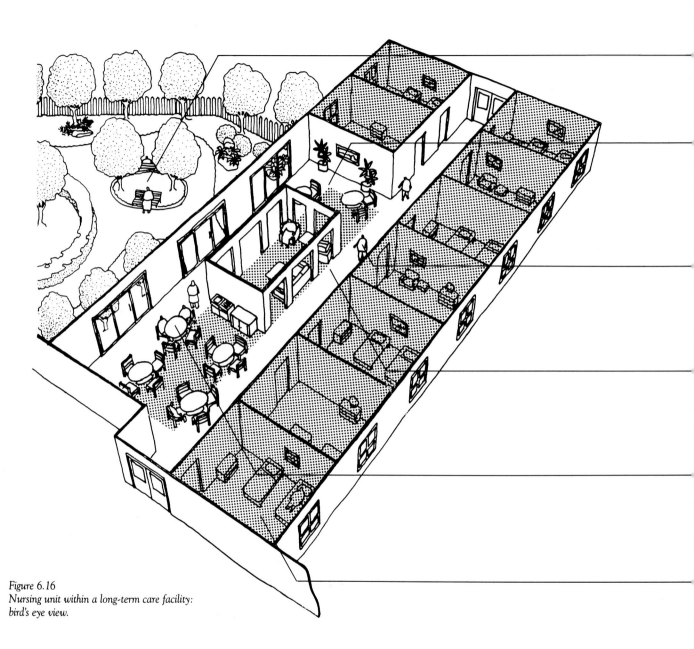

Figure 6.16
Nursing unit within a long-term care facility:
bird's eye view.

Links to the outside
Dining and activity areas have direct access to protected outdoor space.

Clustering activities and spaces (fig. 6.17)
The corridor is interrupted to create social spaces that support familiar activities (dining, living, den) and to add to the homelike ambience. These spaces provide residents with opportunities for privacy or interaction.

Opportunities for meaningful wandering
A walking path extends to a secure outdoor area and links key social spaces indoors.

Sensory stimulation without stress (fig. 6.18)
Partial walls provide a sense of enclosure and security as well as views of activities in adjacent areas and the corridor.

Intimate dining
A clearly identifiable space for dining and an adjoining kitchenette for food preparation and related activities are provided within the unit.

Resident rooms
Although two residents continue to share a room, newly created social spaces serve as places for privacy and reflection.

Figure 6.17
Living and dining areas constitute both the phys-
ical and the functional center of the facility and
the focus of activities.

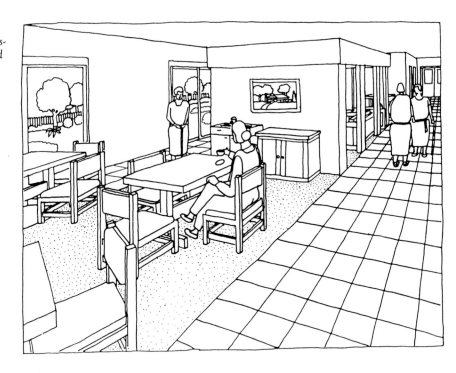

Figure 6.18
The institutional corridor is interrupted by
creating a social space (including dining and
living areas) on one side of the corridor, with
resident rooms arranged in a regular grid on the
other side.

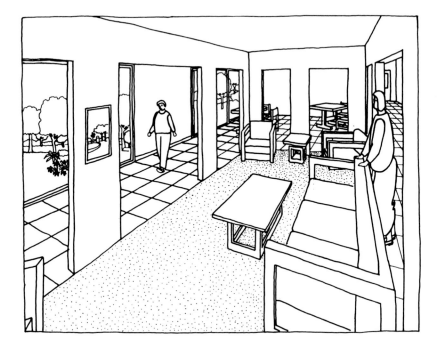

In certain cases, constraints of site or program may make it necessary to accommodate significantly larger numbers of residents in one building. Other situations may also require changing occupancy programs. This scheme, therefore, is designed to function as either a single or a multistory building. It could potentially accommodate not only Alzheimer's care but also hospice, assisted living, group living, and conventional apartments. Achieving such flexibility does necessitate a larger number of residents per cluster (e.g., eighteen persons), as well as a more traditional building organization—a double-loaded corridor (Fig. 6.19).

6.7 Multistory, Multiuse Facility

Organizational Requirements

* Number of residents: Twelve to eighteen per wing; maximum of thirty-six per floor.

Organizational Structure

* Basic clusters can vary in size to accommodate twelve to eighteen residents; fewer than twelve residents may not be economically feasible, and more than eighteen residents may be therapeutically counterproductive.

* Multistory (five to eight story) versions of this scheme could potentially accommodate many housing options along the continuum of care, including independent apartments, group and assisted living, day care, and hospice care, as well as one or more Alzheimer's units.

General Attributes

* While the overall building form is large and somewhat institutional in character, corridors within each wing remain as short as possible and public spaces have direct access to the exterior.

* The location of the Alzheimer's unit on the first floor maximizes potential access to the exterior and minimizes elevator usage.

Building Organization

* Central core functions (kitchen, receiving area, storage, staff retreat area) are located at the center of each floor, conveniently serving both clusters.

* V-shaped clusters minimize the length of corridors, provide views to the exterior from public spaces, and define two sides of outdoor spaces adjacent to the building.

Program

Figure 6.19
Multi-use facility: bird's eye view.

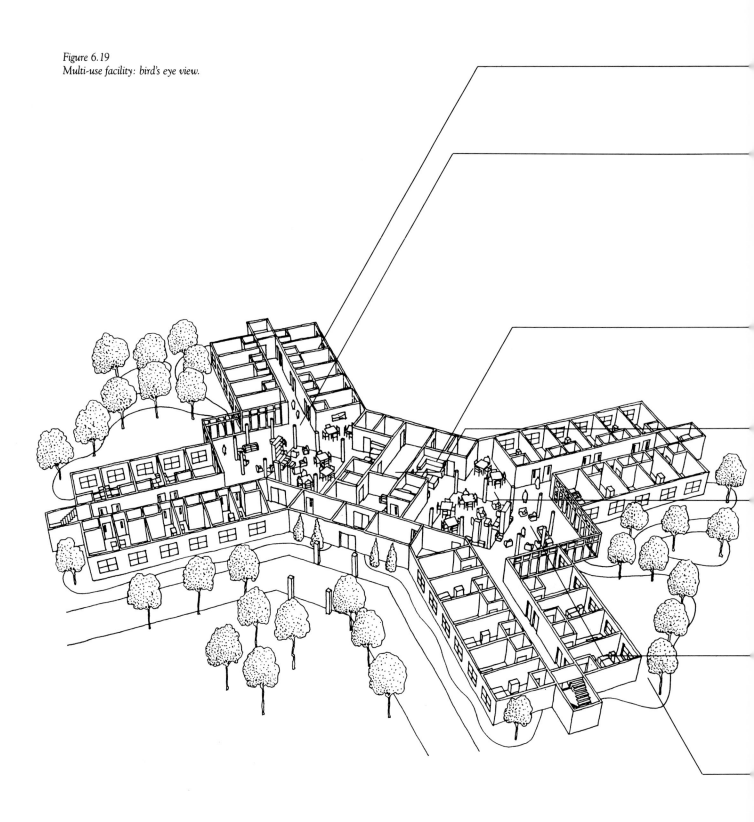

———— Private residents' rooms
Bedrooms provide residents with an opportunity for privacy and solitude.

———— Meaningful wandering path

Assisted bathing room
Bathing facilities are sufficiently large and flexible to allow both assisted and independent bathing and showering.

———— Domestic kitchen
The kitchen is designed and operated to accommodate use by people with dementia, thereby enforcing the homelike nature of the facility.

———— Staff retreat

———— Intimate dining areas

Noninstitutional image/friendly entry
The entry area into the facility reinforces its noninstitutional image.

———— Small activity clusters
Separate activity areas (i.e., dining, living, and activity spaces within the large public zone) are defined and differentiated by columns, different floor finishes, and groupings of furnishings.

———— Positive outdoor space
The shape of the building defines a sheltered outdoor area, accessible from the first-floor Alzheimer's facility.

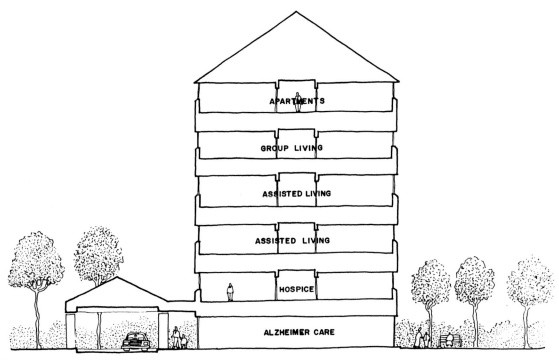

Figure 6.20
Each wing is organized around a set of common spaces that accommodate sitting, dining, and activity areas, as well as physical and/or visual access to the outdoors.

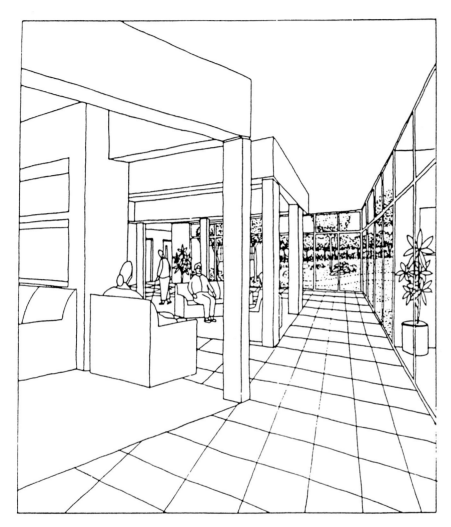

Figure 6.21
Even in multi-story configurations, the relatively
short wings are meant to retain a residential
rather than an institutional quality. The
V-shaped configuration of the building also
serves to define a protected outdoor space at the
ground level.

Overleaf: Hanson Graphic; photograph courtesy of American Medical Services, Inc., photographed by Walter Sheffer and Sue Bartfield

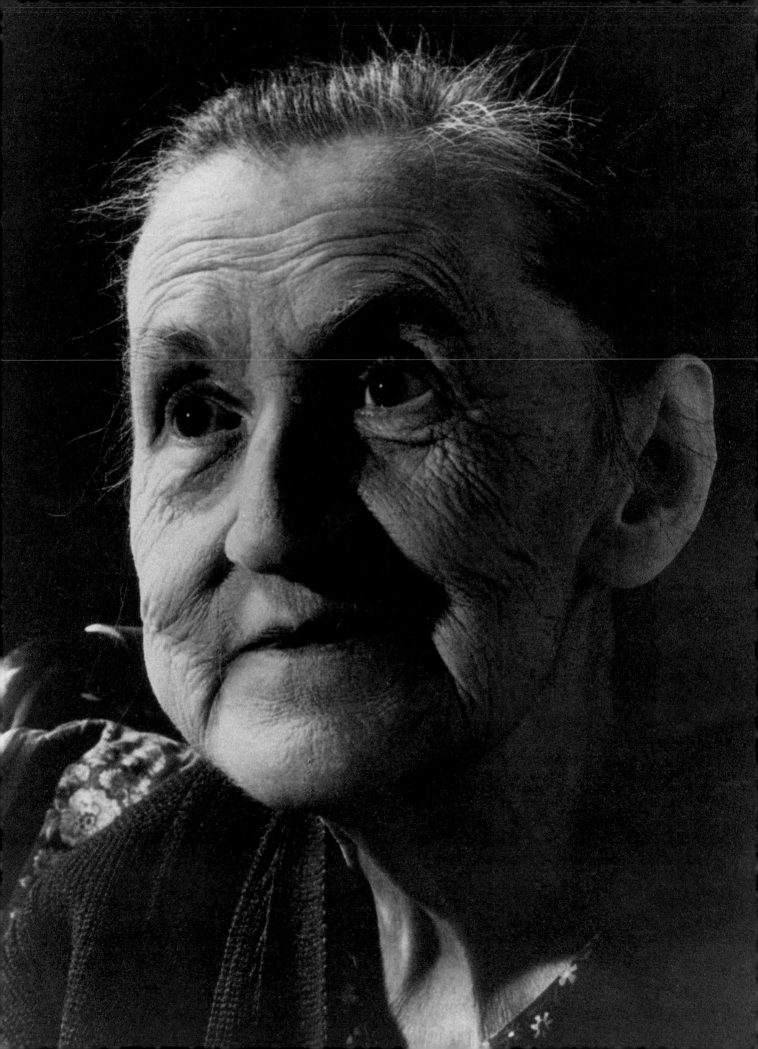

7 Evaluation of the Environment

Building occupancy and use should not be viewed as the termination of the facility development process; rather, it represents a beginning, as people move in and patterns of behavior within the facility are established. At this stage, users may begin to recognize problems or incongruencies among desired programs and goals, architectural features and characteristics, and the resultant performance of the facility. This is an appropriate time to initiate a more formal evaluation of the facility to identify problems, derive lessons, and initiate design responses through either renovation or redesign.

Evaluation may be utilized in three different ways: (1) in a systematic postoccupancy evaluation of an existing facility, (2) as design reviews by architects and clients during the planning and design of new or renovated facilities, and (3) as a stimulus to the thinking of facility administrators, care providers, and designers regarding the untapped therapeutic potential within their own facilities.

The organization of the following evaluation questions corresponds to that of the principles for planning and design presented in chapters 2 to 5, with each set of questions preceded by a brief review of the problem. The intent of this section is to enable those engaged in the planning, design, and operation of facilities for people with dementia to evaluate their setting in terms of general attributes of the environment, issues of building organization, and qualities of activity space.

Environmental options for people with dementia range from the familiar single-family home to the traditional long-term care setting. There is a need for facilities and services that can expand this continuum and create new options for people with dementia and their caregivers. In keeping with the theme of *Holding On to Home*, it is imperative to enhance the domestic and residential nature of all environmental options.

- Does your facility provide for people at different stages of dementia with differing levels of capability? If so, do both organizational policy and the designed environment respond to these differences?

- Is there a range of services for residents of varying functional capabilities?

- Does your facility encourage grouping of residents on the basis of functional level or stage of the disease? How?

- Could your facility offer additional options along the continuum of care, ranging from day care to long-term care?

Questions for Evaluation

2.1 Responsive Continuum of Care

2.2 Tapping Local Resources

Environments for people with dementia need not be self-sufficient; many services available in the community can be utilized by resourceful caregivers and staff members, including use of local health care facilities to replace in-house medical staff and part-time specialist consultants (e.g., music director, craft director) instead of full-time staff specialists. In some instances, community activities and events can serve as sources of recreation for residents (e.g., a local theater troupe might give regular performances, local music groups might be brought in as an occasional activity).

- Of what services in your community might you take advantage? To what extent do you currently utilize these services? For example, does your local community provide opportunities for resident activities such as visits to beauty salons, restaurants, shows, etc.? Which of these opportunities are you currently utilizing?

- If you are in the process of selecting a site for a facility for people with dementia (e.g., a group home or a long-term care setting), are there local resources available that make one alternate location more desirable than another?

2.3 Appropriate Group Size

Groups may be defined in terms of building organization, staffing, and activities. Functional groups can be created on the basis of staffing ratios, social groups in terms of "households," "families," or "clusters." Both types of groups can be reinforced through the layout of the building.

- Is your resident population subdivided on the basis of any of the above strategies? Which one(s)?

- Do different types of grouping reinforce each other (e.g., do residents grouped into spatial clusters also share daily activities)? How does this work?

- How are spatial and social group development expressed in your facility? What are the architectural design characteristics used to reinforce this grouping?

- If you do not currently structure activities and spaces for small groups of residents, how could this be developed in your facility?

3.1 Noninstitutional Character

Image and architectural character of facilities range along a continuum from single-family house (noninstitutional) to hospital (institutional). Typical elements associated with institutional imagery include large, undifferentiated building form; the use of repetitive standardized elements inside (e.g., traditional institutional furniture and fixtures); long, intimidating institutional corridors; and lack of variety in color schemes and carpeting.

- Where would you place your facility along the continuum from noninstitutional to institutional character? Which particular characteristics lead you to this decision?

- Can you identify any of these institutional elements (or others) within your facility? Which ones?

- Are there noninstitutional furnishings or finishes that might be appropriate substitutions? How might you go about making these changes?

3.2 Eliminating Environmental Barriers

Because people with dementia are likely to have reduced capabilities and competence with regard to mobility, physical dexterity, and cognitive faculties, there is often a need for special features that help them more effectively negotiate the environment. Contrast between walls and floors and between corridors and staircases can provide useful compensation for age-related visual impairments. Redundant cueing is one possible means for accommodating reduced cognitive capabilities (e.g., a facility can use olfactory stimulation and photographs of food to allow residents to easily identify the dining room).

- What features and characteristics of your facility are difficult for your resident population to negotiate? Why is this so?

- Which special features in your facility make it more negotiable by people with dementia? How does this occur?

- Where is redundant cueing used in your facility? How is this done?

- What environmental changes would make your facility easier for residents to negotiate? Specifically, when might redundant cueing be introduced? Where could contrast be used to make the environment easier to negotiate? What steps must be taken to facilitate these modifications?

3.3 Things from the Past

Reminiscence is a valuable therapeutic tool and can serve an important role in the lives of people with dementia. Reminiscing can occur at the level of familiar activities (e.g., cooking, gardening), as well in the physical environment (e.g., allowing clients to bring objects from their past into their new environment).

- Do you presently capitalize on reminiscence as a therapeutic resource in the care of people with dementia? How do you do this? Which specific activities, environmental characteristics, and policies encourage reminiscing among residents?

- Are residents allowed and encouraged to personalize their environment? How?

- How can reminiscing and the use of things from the past be incorporated into your setting? For example, how could you incorporate familiar activities into your facility's daily schedule? What changes must be made to incorporate artifacts from residents' pasts into the environment? For example, would this require a change in organizational policy or a change in the furnishing of residents' rooms to allow space for personal artifacts from home?

3.4 Sensory Stimulation without Stress

People with dementia need environments that provide a manageable level of sensory stimulation. Facilities should strike a balance between sensory overload (such as that caused by loud alarms and intercoms) and deprivation (often the result of such devices as repetitive spaces and monochromatic finishes).

- Does your facility offer an appropriate balance between over- and understimulation for people with dementia? What specific characteristics of the environment lead you to make this decision?

- Does your facility also offer varying levels of stimulation for residents? How is this done?

- Which steps have you taken to reduce extraneous environmental stimuli (e.g., loudspeakers, door alarms, distracting televisions or radios)? How was this managed?

- In what ways might you provide a more appropriate level of sensory stimulation for residents? What modifications could be undertaken to reduce sensory overload and/or alleviate underload? How can variety in environmental stimulation also be ensured?

- In what ways could you reduce extraneous stimuli in the environment to amplify various environmental messages (e.g., through the use of sound absorbing material)?

4.1 Clusters of Small Activity Spaces

In facilities that include residents' rooms, these should be arranged around common, small-scale social spaces to create manageable clusters, households, or families of residents. This arrangement can facilitate resident social interaction and functioning and enhance staff satisfaction as well.

- Is there a center of activity in your facility? What is it? How are the public areas in your facility related or linked to each other?

- Is this center space(s) small scale and oriented toward small groups of residents? What characteristics of the space(s) lead you to make this decision?

- Are activity spaces normally available and equally accessible to all residents?

- Is there variety in the types of spaces provided? How is this achieved?

- How could social spaces at the scale of small households be developed?

4.2 Opportunities for Meaningful Wandering

Wandering, a common behavior among people with dementia, can be viewed as a positive opportunity for exercise and exploration. Although modifications should be undertaken to reduce wandering due to disorientation or confusion, remaining forms of wandering should be made more meaningful, interesting, safe, and legible.

- Does your facility provide a clearly defined and safe place for wandering? Where (or what) is this place? How is it defined?

- Can this path be easily and unobtrusively surveyed by staff members or caregivers? How?

- How much of residents' wandering in your facility could be due to disorientation or confusion? How could you discover this?

- Does the wandering path allow visual access to interesting activities and spaces? How does it do this?

- Is this path adjacent to activity areas that might spark client curiosity and invite participation? Does it do this successfully? What leads you to make this evaluation?

- If your facility or home does not currently provide an appropriate area for wandering, how might such a place be created?

- How could the environment be modified to support meaningful wandering behavior and to decrease incidences of wandering due to disorientation or confusion?

4.3 Positive Outdoor Spaces

Attractive and safe outdoor places for people with dementia can provide necessary stimulation and can function as sites for meaningful and familiar activities. Views to the outside will also increase residents' orientation to time, place, and season and can enhance the familiarity and attractiveness of the environment.

- Is an outdoor activity area that is safe and accessible for resident use available at your facility?

- Are interesting and familiar activities incorporated into this space? How?

- Where in your facility are outdoor views provided for residents? Are these views interesting and varied?

- What type of seating is provided in your outdoor area? Where is it located within this space?

- Could an outdoor activity area be developed for your facility if one does not already exist? Which familiar and interesting activities might be incorporated into this space?

- If your facility has an existing outdoor area that is accessible to people with dementia, what are the most significant improvements that could be made to utilize this outdoor space to its fullest potential?

4.4 Other Living Things

The lives of people with dementia can be greatly enriched through the incorporation of plants and animals, which can enhance residents' sense of responsibility and their perception of the environment as homelike and familiar. Flowers, greenhouses, birdfeeders, mini-zoos, and household pets all represent potential means of increasing residents' interaction with other living things.

- How are plants and animals currently being incorporated into the design and activities of your facility?

- How are living things being used to encourage a sense of responsibility and autonomy for the people with dementia with whom you work?

- How could the programs and activities of your facility be changed to offer more opportunities for interaction with other living things?

- How can the design or furnishing of your facility be changed to accommodate more easily the introduction of other living things?

4.5 Public to Private Realms

Like other people, people with dementia need to be provided with access to both public and private places, the use of which will depend upon mood, ongoing activity, etc. Facilities should acknowledge their residents' varying moods and dispositions and provide appropriate and supportive spaces.

- Does your facility provide a range of spaces for communal activities and solitude? For public and private activities? How?

- Are spaces available that support these varying needs of residents? Which spaces are these?

- Could your setting be enhanced to extend this variation of spaces?

5.1 Entry and Transition

The entry area represents the initial introduction to a facility for people with dementia, their caregivers, staff, and visitors. It is therefore imperative that the entry area be friendly and inviting, safe, and easily supervised. It should be somewhat buffered to ensure that entering and exiting do not interrupt ongoing activity; at the same time, the layout of the environment should be easy to understand, for example, by providing a clear overview of the facility from the transition area just outside the entry.

- Is the entry into your facility direct and accessible for both visitors and residents? Is it sheltered from inclement weather and convenient for drop-off (if this is a critical activity)? How is this done?

- If your setting includes individual units or households, is the entry into these areas direct and accessible? Is it easily identifiable to residents, visitors, and staff members? How is this achieved?

- Do entries help or hinder residents' and visitors' sense of orientation? How?

- Are the entry and transition areas in your facility friendly and familiar in nature? How is this impression given?

- How can the entry area into your facility be improved? Can entering and wayfinding in your facility be made more direct and easier to understand? How can the entry area become more reassuring?

- How can entering and leaving become less of an intrusion into on-going activities? Which changes would make the exit from your facility less tempting to wandering residents?

Because people with dementia often display a great deal of passive, "null" be-havior, interesting and attractive social spaces should be provided to encour-age interaction and activity. These spaces should be domestic and familiar in size and scale, furnishings and finishes, and function.

5.2 Shared Spaces

- What are the common social spaces that are available to people with dementia in your facility?

- Are these spaces domestic and familiar in scale and ambience? What characteristics of the environment influence your evaluation?

- How are the common spaces in your facility arranged?

- Is there a variety in the types of spaces available to residents (e.g., in size, function, and character)? How is this provided? Are there pro-visions for social spaces for the entire facility, as well as for small "family" groups? Which spaces are these?

- How could small-scale social spaces be created in your facility? How could existing and new social spaces be more clearly linked to each other?

- How might variety in social spaces be enhanced (e.g., what changes in furnishings and finishes or in function of spaces might provide more variety?)

Domestic, small-scale, residential kitchen facilities can serve as the site for meaningful activity and experiences for people with dementia. Residents' safety when using such spaces must be considered, but concern over potential safety issues should not deter the provision of such spaces. They can be ex-tremely reassuring to residents and may increase their sense of autonomy and control in a significant way.

5.3 Domestic Kitchens

- Does your facility currently have a kitchen area that can be used by people with dementia? Is it safe and accessible? Can it be used independently by residents?

- Is this kitchen domestic in nature? What features or characteristics contribute to this evaluation?

- What types of activities occur in this area? Are these familiar and meaningful activities for your residents?

- What changes is furnishings, finishes, or activities might make this kitchen area more familiar and easier for residents to use and enjoy?

- If there is not presently such a kitchen area in your facility, how could one be created?

5.4 Intimate Dining

Dining can be an important activity for people with dementia, serving to increase their autonomy and independence and their link to healthy and familiar experiences from the past. For this reason, dining should be structured for enjoyment in small, intimate groups. Opportunities for choice in time and place of eating, as well as some decision making in menu, are examples of ways that dining can achieve these goals.

- How is dining structured in your facility? Do all residents eat at the same time in the same place?

- Are residents allowed choice and autonomy in dining (e.g., time or place of dining, decision about what to eat)? How?

- Is dining a pleasant and meaningful activity for residents? What leads you to make this evaluation?

- How could more intimate dining be provided (e.g., smaller places or smaller groups for dining) in your facility? What changes might be made to provide residents greater flexibility in seating or in deciding what or when to eat?

5.5 Activity Alcoves

The incorporation of small activity alcoves will reinforce small group activities; they can serve as sites for visiting, intimate socialization, and resident retreat and reflection. These places should be designed to provide closure and will be especially successful when they overlook adjacent activities and give a sense of the activities and functions that they house.

- Other than resident rooms and large common areas, does your facility have clearly defined small social spaces for resident use? What are these?

- Are these spaces adjacent to circulation paths or activity areas to encourage resident observation of ongoing activities? Are they successful in encouraging this?

- Do these activity alcoves also provide opportunities for quiet reminiscence and retreat? How is this done?

- Do these spaces function as landmarks, facilitating orientation and wayfinding? How do they do this?

- How could such activity alcoves be introduced or improved in your facility?

When possible, resident rooms should function as fundamentally private spaces, in keeping with the traditional and familiar associations of "bedroom." Although some residents may choose to engage in social activities in their rooms, these should not be the only spaces available for social activities, such as visiting.

- Are residents' rooms in your facility treated as essentially private spaces (in terms of function and ambience)? How is this achieved?

- How are residents' rooms furnished? Are they domestic and familiar in appearance and ambience? What characteristics contribute to this quality?

- Do residents' rooms also function as small-scale social spaces in your facility? If so, how could this function be transferred elsewhere in the facility?

- Can residents' rooms have stronger associations to that with which residents are most familiar (e.g., a domestic appearance and function)? In what ways can the privacy of residents' rooms be enhanced?

Bathing is often a difficult and frightening experience for people with dementia. However, it can also offer a chance to exercise autonomy and independence. Environmental modifications (e.g., grab bars, sloped-floor showers with no lip, the development of private areas for bathing or showering) should be undertaken to ensure residents' privacy and autonomy to the greatest extent possible.

- Does your facility provide bathing and/or showering facilities for use by people with dementia?

- What type of equipment and furnishings do residents presently use for bathing and/or showering? Are bathing facilities domestic in nature and familiar to residents?

- What portion of the people with dementia in your facility presently shower or bath independently or with minimal staff assistance? Do bathing equipment and policies in your setting encourage independent bathing by people with dementia? How (e.g., are they accessible for use without assistance?)

- What types of familiar and accessible bathing furnishings (e.g., a shower with no lip that is wheelchair-accessible) might replace frightening institutional contraptions (e.g., hydraulic lifts into deep bathtubs) in your facility?

- If your facility does not presently offer bathing and grooming services to assist elderly caregivers of people with dementia, might this be incorporated into the services offered by your facility (i.e., in the case of day care centers)?

• What environmental modifications and policy changes might increase the percentage of residents in your facility who are able to bathe independently?

5.8 Independent Toileting

Incontinence, often associated with advancing dementia, can be devastating to the person with Alzheimer's disease. In addition, even among continent residents, toileting is often less than private and independently managed. All possible measures should be undertaken to enhance independent toileting for all persons with dementia. Such measures might include designing toileting areas that are private yet quickly located and easily identified.

• Are toileting areas in your home or facility accessible to and independently usable by people with dementia?

• Are they easy to locate and to identify?

• Do toileting areas ensure privacy for residents? How? If your facility includes resident rooms, are these associated with private toileting areas for the residents of each room?

• What modifications (e.g., the addition of grab bars, the use of a raised toilet seat) would make toileting areas easier for residents to use independently?

• Where group toileting areas (restrooms for more than one person) are already in place in your facility, what design changes (e.g., the addition of doors to toilet stalls) can increase privacy for residents?

• How can toileting areas in your facility be modified to be easier for residents to locate and identify?

5.9 Places for Visiting

Residents of facilities for people with dementia can benefit greatly by visits from family members and friends. In addition, visiting is an important activity for caregivers. It should, therefore, be accommodated by providing interesting, reassuring, and noninstitutional areas for visiting, preferably located adjacent to activities and artifacts that might make visiting a more positive experience.

• Where in your facility do residents currently visit with family members or friends?

• Do these spaces encourage conversation and meaningful interaction with residents? How?

• Are these spaces domestic and familiar in nature, to reassure family members and friends and encourage them to visit and to participate in the care of the resident? What characteristics create this feeling?

• How could new spaces be developed or existing spaces be enhanced to allow greater privacy during visiting? How can visiting areas become more friendly and residential in character?

Staff members occasionally need a space in which to "retreat" from contact with clients or to take short breaks.

- Do staff in your facility currently have a place for such retreat?

- Is there a place where staff members can complete required work tasks, have a cup of coffee, or hold private conversations free from distraction by residents or family members? How does this space meet these staff needs?

- Where such a space does not exist, how could a staff retreat area be developed or enhanced to address these needs?

5.10 Staff Retreat

Overleaf: Hanson Graphic; photograph courtesy of American Medical Services, Inc., photographed by Walter Sheffer and Sue Bartfield

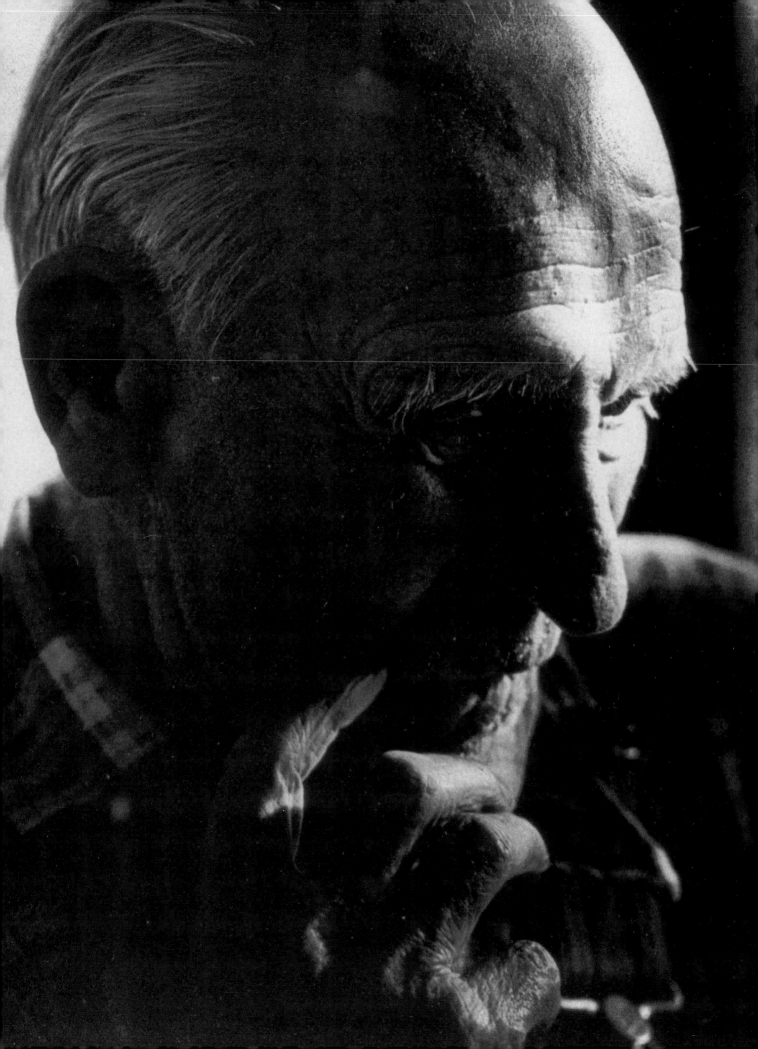

References

Alexander, C. (1969). *Notes on the synthesis of form.* Cambridge, Mass: Harvard University Press.

Alverman, M. (1979). Towards improving geriatric care with environmental interventions emphasizing a home like atmosphere: An environmental experience. *Journal of Gerontological Nursing, 5* (3), 13–17.

American Institute of Architects. (1971). *Statement of the architect's services.* Washington, D.C.: American Institute of Architects.

Andreason, M. (1985). Make a safe environment by design. *Journal of Gerontological Nursing, II* (6), 18–22.

Barnes, J. (1974). Effects of reality orientation classroom on memory loss, confusion, and disorientation in geriatric patients. *Gerontologist, 14,* 138–142.

Benson, D., Cameron, D., Humbach, E., Servino, L., and Gambert, S. (1987). Establishment and impact of a dementia unit within a nursing home. *American Geriatrics Society, 35* (4), 320–323.

Brill, M., Margulis, S., Konar, E., and BOSTI. (1984). *Using office design to increase productivity,* Vol. 1. Buffalo, N.Y.: Workplace Design and Productivity.

Calkins, M. (1986). *A design guide for special care units for people with Alzheimer's disease and related disorders.* Master of Architecture thesis, School of Architecture and Urban Planning, University of Wisconsin-Milwaukee.

Calkins, M. (1987). Designing special care units: A systematic approach. *American Journal of Alzheimer's Care and Research, 2,* 2–3.

Calkins, M. (1988). *Design for dementia: Planning environments for the elderly and confused.* Owings Mills, Md.: National Health Publishing.

Cohen, U., Weisman, G., Ray, K., Rand, J., and Toyne, R. (1988). *Alzheimer's disease and environmental design: Case studies.* Washington, D.C.: Health Facilities Research Program, AIA/ACSA Council on Architectural Research.

Coons, D. (1985). Alive and well at Wesley Hall. *Quarterly: A Journal of Long Term Care, 21,* (2), 10–14.

Coons, D. (1987). Designing a residential care unit for persons with dementia. Washington, D.C.: U.S. Congress, Office of Technology Assessment.

Coons, D. (1988). Wandering. *American Journal of Alzheimer's Care and Related Disorders and Research, 3* (1), 31–36.

Coons, D., and Spencer, B. (1983). The older person's response to therapy: A. The in-hospital therapeutic community. *Psychiatric Quarterly, 55* (2&3), 156–172.

DeLong, A. J. (1970). The microspatial structure of the older person. In L. A. Pastalan and D. H. Carson (eds.), *The spatial behavior of older people.* Ann Arbor: Institute of Gerontology, University of Michigan.

Folsom, J. (1983). Reality orientation. In B. Reisberg (ed.), *Alzheimer's disease: The standard reference* (pp. 449–454). New York: Free Press.

Fraser, D. (1978). Behavioral effects of environmental changes among a psychiatric geriatric population. Pilot Project 2. Norristown State Hospital Psychology Department, Norristown, Pa.

Gifford, R. (1987). *Environmental psychology.* Newton, Mass.: Allyn and Bacon.

Gilleard, C. (1984). *Living with dementia: Community care of the elderly mentally infirm.* Philadelphia: Charles Press.

Glaser, B., and Strass, H. (1968). Time for dying. *Journal of Family Practice, 12,* 831–837.

Gnaedinger, N. (1989). *Housing Alzheimer's disease at home.* Ottawa: External Research Program, Canada Mortgage and Housing Corporation.

Goffman, E. (1961). *Asylums: Essays on the social situation of mental patients and other inmates.* Garden City, N.Y.: Anchor.

References

Goldsmith, S. (1976). *Designing for the disabled.* London: Royal Institute of British Architects.

Gottesman, L. E., and Bourestom, N. C. (1974). Why nursing homes do what they do. *Gerontologist, 14,* 501–506.

Green, L. (1987). *Designing the physical environment for persons with dementia: An audiovisual production. User's manual.* Ann Arbor: Regents of the University of Michigan.

Greene, V. L., and Monahan, D. J. (1982). The impact of visitation on patient well-being in nursing homes. *Gerontologist, 22,* 410–423.

Gubrium, J. (1986). Oldtimers and Alzheimer's disease: The descriptive organization of senility. Greenwich, Conn.: Jai Press.

Gwyther, L. (1986). Treating behavior as a symptom of illness. *Provider,* May, 18–21.

Hall, G., and Buckwalter, K. (1986). *Progressively lowered stress threshold: A conceptual model for care of adults with Alzheimer's disease.* Paper presented at the annual meeting of the American Association of Neurosciences Nurses, April 15, 1986, Denver, Colo.

Harris, H., Lipman, A., and Slater, R. (1977). Architectural design: The spatial location and interactions of old people. *Gerontology, 23,* 390–400.

Heston, L., and White, J. (1983). *Dementia: a practical guide to Alzheimer's disease and related illnesses.* New York: W. H. Freeman and Co.

Hiatt, L. (1981). Designing therapeutic dining. *Nursing Homes,* April/May, 33–39.

Hofland, B. (1988). Autonomy in long term care: Background issues and a progammatic response. *Gerontologist, 28 (Suppl.),* 3–9.

Howell, S. (1980). *Designing for aging: Patterns of use.* Cambridge, Mass.: MIT Press.

Hussian, R., and Brown, D. (1987). Use of two-dimensional grid patterns to limit hazardous ambulation in demented patients. *Journal of Gerontology, 42* (5), 558–560.

Hyde, J. (1989). The physical environment and the care of Alzheimer's patients: An experiential survey of Massachusetts' Alzheimer's units. *American Journal of Alzheimer's Care and Related Disorders and Research, 4* (3), 36–44.

Kahn, R. (1975). The mental health system and the future aged. *Gerontologist, 16 (Suppl),* 24–31.

Kelly, W. (ed.). (1984). *Alzheimer's disease and related disorders: Research and management.* Springfield, Ill.: Charles C Thomas.

Kirk, S., Eichinger, C., and Spreckelmeyer, K. (1984). In G. S. Lasdon and J. S. Gann (eds.), *The future of hospital design.* Washington, D.C.: U.S. Department of Health and Human Services.

Koncelik, J. (1976). *Designing the open nursing home.* Stroudsburg, Pa.: Dowden, Hutchinson, and Ross, Inc.

Koncelik, J. (1979). Human factors and environmental design for the aging: Aspects of physiological change and sensory loss as design criteria. In T. Byerts, S. Howell, and L. Pastalan (eds.), *Environmental context of aging* (pp. 107–117). New York: Garland STPM.

Kromm, D., and Kromm, Y. (1985). A nursing home designed for Alzheimer's disease patients at Newton Presbyterian Manor. *Nursing Homes,* May/June, 30–31.

Lang, J. (1987). *Creating architectural theory: The role of the behavioral sciences in environmental design.* New York: Van Nostrand Reinhold.

Langer, E., and Rodin, J. (1976). The effects of choice and enhanced personal responsibility for the aged: A field experiment in an institutional setting. *Journal of Personality and Social Psychology, 34,* 191–198.

Lawton, M. P. (1970). Ecology and aging. In L. Pastalan and D. A. Carson (eds.),

Spatial behavior of older people. Ann Arbor: Institute of Gerontology, University of Michigan.

Lawton, M. P. (1981). Sensory deprivation and the effect of the environment on management of the patient with senile dementia. In N. Miller and G. Cohen (eds.), *Clinical aspects of Alzheimer's disease and senile dementia* (pp. 251-271). New York: Raven Press.

Lawton, M. P. (1987). Environmental approaches to research and treatment of Alzheimer's disease. In E. Light and B. Liebowitz (eds.), *Alzheimer's disease, treatment, and family stress: Directions for research.* Washington, D.C.: National Institute of Mental Health.

Lawton, M. P., Fulcomer, M., and Kleban, M. (1984). Architecture for the mentally impaired elderly. *Environment and Behavior, 16,* 730–757.

Lawton, M. P., Leibowitz, B., and Charon, H. (1970). Physical structure and the behavior of senile patients following ward remodeling. *Aging and human development, 1,* 231–239.

Lawton, M. P., and Nahemow, L. (1973). Ecology and the aging process. In C. Eisdorfer and M. P. Lawton (eds.), *Psychology of adult development and aging.* Washington, D.C.: American Psychological Association.

Laxton, C. (1985). The John D. French Center for Alzheimer's disease. *Caring.* Dec., 22–24.

Liebowitz, B., Lawton, M. P., and Waldman, A. (1979). Evaluation: Designing for confused elderly people. *American Institute of Architects Journal, 68,* 59–61.

Lindeman, D. (1984). *Alzheimer's disease handbook.* San Francisco: Aging Health Policy Center. Grant No. 90-AP0003.

Lowenthal, M., Berkman, P., and associates (1967). *Aging and mental disorder in San Francisco.* San Francisco: Jossey-Bass.

Mace, N. (1987). Programs and services which specialize in the care of persons with dementing illnesses—issues and options. *American Journal of Alzheimer's Care and Research,* May/June, 10–17.

Mace, N., and Rabins, P. (1981). *The 36 hour day.* Baltimore: Johns Hopkins University Press.

Matthew, L., Sloan, P., Kilby, M., and Flood, R. (1988). What's different about a special care unit for dementia patients: A comparative study. *American Journal of Alzheimer's and Related Disorders Care and Research, 3* (2), 16–23.

Moos, R., and Lemke, S. (1980). Assessing the physical and architectural features of sheltered care settings. *Journal of Gerontology, 35* (4), 571–583.

Moos, R., and Lemke, S. (1984). Supportive residential settings for older people. In I. Altman and M. Lawton (eds.), *Elderly people and their environments* (pp. 159–190). New York: Plenum.

Namazi, K., Rosner, T., and Calkins, M. (1989). Visual barriers to prevent ambulatory Alzheimer's patients from exiting through an emergency door. *Gerontologist, 29,* 699–702.

National Advisory Council on Aging, Government of Canada (1987). *Housing an aging population: Guidelines for development and design.* Ottawa: Minister of Supply and Services.

Nelson, M., and Paluck, R. (1980). Territorial markings, self-concept, and mental status of the institutionalized elderly. *Gerontologist, 20* (1), 96–98.

Ohta, R., and Ohta, B. (1988). Special care units for Alzheimer's disease patients: A critical look. *Gerontologist, 28* (6), 803–808.

Pastalan, L. (1979). Sensory changes and environmental behaviors. In T. Byerts, S. Howell, and L. Pastalan (eds.), *Environmental context of aging* (pp. 118–126). New York: Garland STPM.

Peppard, N. (1986). Effective design of special care units. *Provider,* May, 14–17.

Peterson, R. F., Knapp, T. J., Rosen, J. C., and Pither, B. F. (1977). The effects of furniture arrangement on the behavior of geriatric patients. *Behavior Therapy, 8,* 464–467.

Pynoos, J., and Ohta, R. (1988). *Home environment management for Alzheimer's care givers: a program of research and dissemination to reduce burden and increase safety and functioning.* Los Angeles: University of Southern California, AARP Andrus Foundation.

Pynoos, J., and Stacey, C. (1986). Specialized facilities for senile dementia patients. In M. Gilhooly, S. Zarit, and J. Birren (eds.), *The dementias: Policy and management.* Englewood Cliffs, N.J.: Prentice-Hall.

Rabins, P. (1982). The impact of dementia of the family. *Journal of the American Medical Association, 248* (3), 333–335.

Rand, J., Steiner, V., Toyne, R., Cohen, U., and Weisman, G. (1987). *Environments for people with dementia: Annotated bibliography.* Washington, D.C.: Health Facilities Research Program, AIA/ACSA Council on Architectural Research.

Rapelje, D., Papp, P., and Crawford, L. (1981). Creating a therapeutic park for the mentally frail. *Dimensions in health service,* Sept., 12–14.

Rapelje, D., Papp, P., and Crawford, L. (no date). *A therapeutic park for mentally frail residents of an Ontario Home for Senior Citizens.* Welland, Ont.: Regional Senior Citizens' Department.

Regnier, V. (1985). *Behavioral and environmental aspects of outdoor space use in housing for the elderly.* Los Angeles: Andrus Gerontology Center.

Reisberg, B. (1983). An overview of current concepts of Alzheimer's disease, senile demenia and age-associated cognitive decline. In B. Reisberg (ed.), *Alzheimer's disease: The standard reference* (pp. 6–20). New York: Free Press.

Roach, M. (1984). Reflections in a fake mirror. *Discover, 8,* 76–85.

Rostenberg, W. (1986) *Design planning for freestanding ambulatory care facilities: A primer for health care providers and architects.* Chicago: American Hospital Publishing.

Sands, D., and Suzuki, T. (1983). Adult day care for Alzheimer's patients and their familires. *Gerontologist, 23* (1), 21–23.

Shamoian, C. (1984). *Biology and treatment of dementia in the elderly.* Washington, D.C.: American Psychiatric Press.

Shumaker, S., and Pequegnat, W. (1989). Hospital design, health providers, and the delivery of effective health care. In E. H. Zube and G. T. Moore (eds.), *Advances in environments, behavior, and design,* Vol. 2. New York: Plenum Press.

Snyder. L. (1984). Archetypal place and the needs of the aging. In M. Spivak (ed.), *Institutional settings: An environmental design approach.* New York: Human Sciences Press.

Snyder, L. H., Rupprecht, P., Pyrek, J., Brekhus, S., and Moss, T. (1978). Wandering. *Gerontologist, 18* (3), 272–280.

Sommer, R. (1969). *Personal space: The behavioral basis of design.* Englewood Cliffs, N.J.: Prentice-Hall.

Sommer, R. (1974). *Tight spaces.* Englewood Cliffs, N.J.: Prentice-Hall.

Stahler, G., Frazer, D., and Rappaport, H. (1984). The evaluation of an environmental remodeling program on a psychiatric geriatric ward. *Journal of Social Psychology, 123,* 101–113.

Stevens, P. S. (1987). Design for dementia: Recreating the loving family. *American Journal of Alzheimer's Care and Research,* Jan./Feb., 16–22.

U.S. Congress Office of Technology Assessment (1987). *Losing a million minds: Confronting the tragedy of Alzheimer's disease and other dementias.* (OTA-BA-323). Washington, D.C.: U.S. Government Printing Office.

Verderber, S. (1982). Designing for the therapeutic functions of windows in the hospital rehabilitation environment. In P. Bart, A. Chen, and G. Francescato (eds.), *Knowledge for design.* Washington, D.C.: Environmental Design Research Association.

Weisman, G. (1987). Improving way-finding and architectural legibility in housing for the elderly. In V. Regnier and J. Pynoos (eds.), *Housing for the elderly: Design directives and policy considerations* (pp. 441–464). New York: Elsevier.

Whyte, W. (1980). *The social life of small urban spaces.* Washington, D.C.: Conservation Foundation.

Zeisel, J. (1981). Inquiry by design: Tools for environment-behavior research. Monterey, Calif.: Brooks-Cole.

Zeisel, J., Welch, P., and Demos, S. (1978). *Low rise housing for older people.* Washington, D.C.: Department of Housing and Urban Development.

Index

(Page numbers in italics refer to illustrations or captions.)

Designed by Chris L. Hotvedt.

Composed by Brushwood Graphics, Inc., in Goudy Old Style text and Futura and Goudy Old Style Italic display.

Printed by Thomson-Shore, Inc., on 80-lb. Glatco Matte.